YOUR HEALING MOUTH

Unlocking Ancient Ayurvedic Secrets for Optimal Dental Health

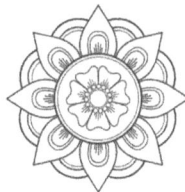

Dr Aushi Patel

BDS (Lond), AIAOMT

The information in this book represents the genuine cultural, lived and professional experience of the author. It is not offered as medical advice nor as a professional service in the treatment of dental conditions, but as a guide to possible avoidance of such conditions through lifestyle choices.

Some of the issues covered by the author challenge the status quo in the dental profession and remain topics of current debate and research. The reader should consult with a relevantly qualified health practitioner before implementing any of the suggestions or products discussed in this book, which are only intended to support the reader as they research how to best enhance their own dental health.

The author's professional anecdotes and references to patient stories are a composite of her clinical experience. They are created by the author for the education and engagement of the reader and do not reference any of the author's specific patient cases.

draushipatel.com

First Edition: January 2024

ISBN: 978-0-6459730-0-6

I dedicate this book to the memory of
my beloved Mumaji

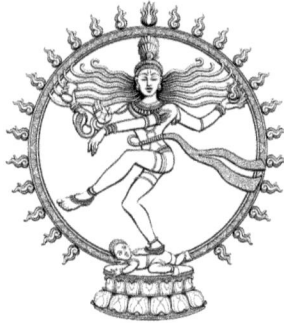

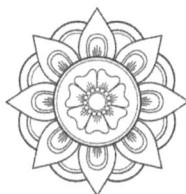

CONTENTS

PREFACE - OPENING TO GREATER WISDOM   vii

PART 1 - YOUR MOUTH IS YOUR FRIEND

CHAPTER 1 - Welcome to a New Way of Looking at Your Mouth - *Your Key to Good Health*   3
CHAPTER 2 - Ayurveda and Dental Health - *How Ancient Wisdom Can Support You*   7

PART 2 - WHAT IS YOUR MOUTH TELLING YOU?

CHAPTER 3 - Gum Disease - *The King of Deception*   29
CHAPTER 4 - Tooth Decay - *There's More to Preventing Cavities than Brushing and Flossing*   49
CHAPTER 5 - Stressed-Out Mouth - *Clenching and Grinding: The Burden Our Teeth Bear*   69

PART 3 - YOUR NEW RELATIONSHIP WITH YOUR MOUTH

CHAPTER 6 - From Mundane to Enjoyable - *Turn Your Daily Dental Routine into a Beautiful, Nourishing Ritual*   89

EPILOGUE - IF IT'S IN YOUR MOUTH, IT'S IN YOUR BODY   109

APPENDIX A - Ayurveda Dosha Quiz   111
APPENDIX B - Resources   123
Endnotes   125
Acknowledgements   141
About the Author   143
Anokhi Veda Ayurvedic Oral Care   145
Index   149

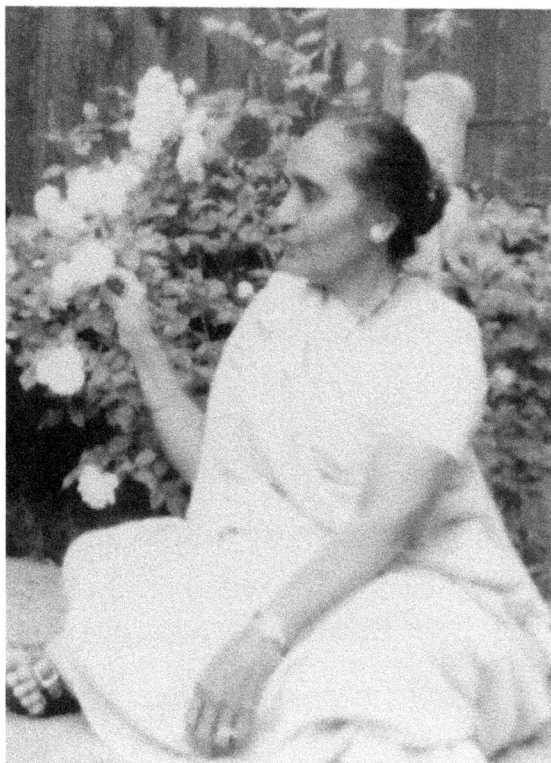

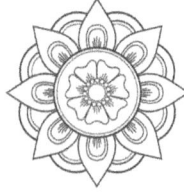

OPENING TO GREATER WISDOM

For three days, I sat with my beloved grandmother as she lay in her hospital bed in North London. I brushed her hair and sang mantras to her just as she had to me from the day I was born.

As I held her warm, soft hand in mine, I was overwhelmed with a deep sense of love and gratitude for this strong, divine woman who had played such a special role in shaping my life. These feelings eclipsed the underlying sorrow that would soon burst forth with her inevitable passing.

My grandmother was given the name Kamla, which in Sanskrit, the ancient language of India, means 'lotus'. Nevertheless, all her grandchildren called her 'Mumaji'. She was my rock and my anchor.

A couple of years after I was born, our family and other Indians who called Uganda home were forced into exile. We initially moved to London, where Mumaji took me under her wing.

She buffered the turmoil and trauma we went through, the extreme disorientation, by holding me on her lap and telling me stories about the mythological gods and goddesses of our rich Vedic culture. This is one of my fondest, most treasured memories. She taught me to sing Sanskrit mantras before I could even speak English!

True to her birth name, my grandmother embodied the expression 'from the mud grows the lotus'. She was born in a small village in India and experienced trauma from a young age when her mother passed away. She was only four years old and was brought up by her relatives. When she was sixteen, she married my grandfather, a man she deeply respected and loved. Soon after, they moved from India to Uganda, where she had to adapt to her new life in East Africa. She soon settled in and went on to bear seven children, my mother being one of them.

Shortly before we were exiled, my grandfather passed away, leaving my grandmother a widow at a young age. As always, she was willing to meet life as it came. She carried her grief with her when we moved, and despite the additional hardship of being displaced to another country, she rose to the occasion, relying on her ability to find the light in the darkness and transform the mud into the lotus. She accepted what life gave her with humility and gratitude, yet always carried an inner fire.

Mumaji's deep connection to the divine gave her a mystical aura, a grace and beauty in everything she encountered. She was dedicated to embracing the devotional practices and Ayurvedic teachings she had learnt growing up in India.

In her home, her pride and joy was her temple shrine filled with small figurines and framed images of various Hindu gods and goddesses. Here she began each day at five a.m. with a devotional ritual by lighting a stick of incense. To this day, the smell of its sweet, perfumed scent takes me back to the memory of her temple. She sang mantras and poured offerings of rose petals and milk over her statues, meditating for at least a couple of hours.

I have memories of my time in her London home before I reached school age, eagerly shadowing her as she went about her daily activities. She had a passion for writing and diligently maintained a notebook brimming with Vedic mantras she sang with joy. Inspired by her devotion, I yearned to be just like her and asked for my very own notebook and a saree so I could join her in the sacred realm of her devotional practice.

When I think back on it, the best way I can describe Mumaji is that she embodied the essence of the Divine Feminine. She was my Shakti; she was my strength.

Growing up, I absorbed and embraced her spiritual values. With each mythological tale she told me, she explained the morals of the story: Be honest, practise forgiveness and lead a heart-centered life. *Seva*, or service, was very important to her, as was *Ahimsa*, to do no harm, which later showed up in my Hippocratic Oath as a dentist.

Dentistry was a calling I'd felt since I was nine years old, when my mother took me to her dental appointment with her youngest brother, a dentist. He was someone I'd always loved and looked up to as a role model.

Although I was supposed to stay in the waiting area, I snuck into the treatment room. The tools and equipment in his workplace captivated me, and once the procedure on my mother began, I was fascinated. At that moment, I knew that when I grew up, I would follow in my uncle's footsteps and become a dentist.

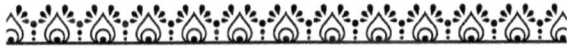

When I think back on it, the best way I can describe Mumaji is that she embodied the essence of the Divine Feminine. She was my Shakti; she was my strength.

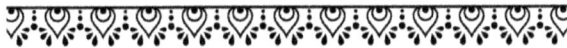

The years passed, and my grandmother and I remained close no matter where I lived. I always admired her deep commitment to serving others and her strong belief that everyone, especially women, had the right to a quality education no matter their life circumstances. Despite Mumaji's limited resources, she made it possible for a number of underprivileged children in India to receive an education. I'm proud to say that many of those students have become successful business leaders in the United States.

So naturally, she was over the moon when I was accepted into the esteemed King's College School of Medicine and Dentistry in London. I can still see her beaming smile and the happiness she radiated when I graduated, earning my degree and the title of Dr Patel.

Her message was crystal clear: Always be humble because you and your hands are channelling divine energy, which is something far greater than you.

Mumaji instilled in me not only her moral values but also gave me my cultural identity. I'm of Indian ancestry but was born in Uganda, as were my parents. Shortly after we were exiled, my parents and I moved to Canada and lived there until I was fourteen. We then relocated to the UK, where I lived for the next fifteen years and completed my education. Today, and for more than two decades, I've called Australia my home. Although I've lived around the world and have been exposed to many cultures, I've never truly felt I belonged anywhere, not even in India, where I'm looked upon as a foreigner!

But Mumaji would have none of it. Once, when I told her how I felt, her eyes flashed with fierceness. What she said gave me roots that served as my anchor. 'You are Indian,' she said, 'and you should be proud.'

I can now appreciate how strong and resilient Mumaji was. She adapted to life in East Africa, learning to speak the native language, Swahili, and then in England, learning to speak English. Yet no matter where she was, she embraced her Indian heritage and wore a saree with pride every day. Because of her, no matter where I might be in the world, I can recite a mantra and find my way back to the home of my heart and soul: my Indian heritage.

The early years of my career in the UK were spent working in National Health Service hospitals, first in paediatric dentistry, and then oral and maxillofacial surgery. Working alongside oncologists, ear, nose and throat surgeons and other medical specialists gave me a deep understanding of how closely the mouth is connected to the rest of the body. As a new graduate, I was already viewing the mouth through a medical lens.

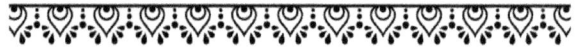

After five years in London, my desire to live closer to the ocean and my love of scuba diving inspired me to relocate to Sydney, Australia. It was here, through a series of predestined events, that I was introduced to the world of holistic dentistry.

Esteemed dentists were recognising the connection between oral health and overall wellbeing, which aligned with the insights I had gained from my previous experience working in hospitals. Moreover, they were offering a more natural approach to dental care, which fit perfectly with my deep-rooted connection to natural healing.

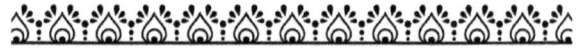

> As a new graduate, I was already viewing the mouth through a medical lens.

As I began my own study and research, I started connecting with other like-minded dentists around the world. My knowledge of the potentially harmful effects of certain dental procedures and materials increased, and I found myself starting to question some of the ways modern dentistry was practised.

At the same time, my eyes were opened to the possibilities of a more conscious and integrative way of offering dental care to my patients. When I graduated, I took the Hippocratic oath of 'premium non nocere', which translates to 'first do no harm'. Now I saw how to take that oath even further. I learned more about the underlying philosophies of holistic dentistry, also known as biological dentistry, which only deepened my understanding of and appreciation for the mouth–body connection.

A desire and a vision began to grow in me: I wanted to change dentistry from its traditional 'drill and fill' method to one that takes a gentler, more wellness-based approach to healing.

With this goal in mind, I founded my Sydney practice, Anokhi Dental. In Sanskrit, the word *anokhi* signifies 'unique'. I would treat each patient as a unique and whole individual. I wanted their healing to begin as soon as they entered my clinic, where they would experience a tranquil, calming environment.

My involvement in my patients' healing was about more than just their teeth. I blended all the aspects of wellbeing I had learnt so I could support their overall health.

This shift in perspective led me to approach everything with fresh eyes, including the issues that presented themselves in my daily dental practice, such as gum disease, decay and teeth grinding.

I recognised the importance of delving deeper and began asking my patients questions such as:

* What did they eat?
* How was their digestion?
* What oral care products were they using?
* Did they breathe through their nose or their mouth?

It was becoming clear to me that the underlying factors contributing to their dental conditions extended beyond the mouth, prompting me to explore the root causes and take a more holistic approach to their oral health.

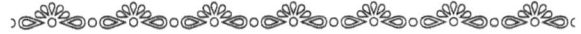

> I blended all the aspects of wellbeing I had learned so I could support their overall health.

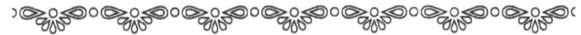

Within the realm of dental treatments, I came to understand that some of the procedures and materials used in modern dentistry, such as fluoride and mercury amalgam were toxic and not supportive of overall health. I consciously chose to avoid those procedures and materials and have done so for more than twenty years.

I knew Mumaji was proud of the work I was doing, but there was more to come. When I received the call that she had suffered a stroke and been admitted to hospital, I rushed from Sydney to London.

At her bedside, I watched her body inhale and exhale, her face at peace as she slept. Then, for just a moment, she opened her grey-blue, ethereal eyes and fixed her gaze on me. Her look shook me to my core. Once again, she closed her eyes, then slipped away from this worldly realm.

To this day, I can't describe the energy in the room that night, except to say I had never felt anything like it before. In that profound moment, a message was being conveyed to me, one whose full meaning I had yet to fully grasp and comprehend.

When I returned home to Sydney after her passing, I was in a daze for weeks. I spoke with my trusted healer about my loss and began processing my grief. He explained that when my grandmother looked into my eyes, at that precise moment she passed to me 'the ball of wisdom'. My grandmother was indeed a wise woman, no doubt about it. What had she imparted to me?

A few months later, the answer would begin to be unveiled. Circumstances with the pandemic forced me to temporarily close my clinic, and after several decades dedicated to my dental practice, I suddenly had time on my hands for personal study.

I welcomed this opening as an opportunity to learn more about Ayurveda, a practice my grandmother had subtly exposed me to from a very young age without my even knowing it. A trip to India early in my career, which you'll read about later, sparked my interest in Ayurveda, and I've been carrying the desire to learn more about it ever since. I started my study under the guidance of a Western-trained medical doctor with a special interest in Ayurveda. Eventually, I earned a certificate in Ayurvedic healing.

It was during this time that I began to more fully appreciate my grandmother's deep knowledge of health and how she related to the natural world.

In many respects, Mumaji had served as her own physician and healer. She had a natural remedy for nearly every ailment, and most of the ingredients – herbs and spices – were already in her kitchen. She lived by herself in her own home quite independently until just days before she passed away.

Mumaji was ninety-eight. She had lived a full life. The hospital staff were amazed at how healthy she had been up to that point and what little medication she'd been taking.

Without realising it, I had been immersed in the traditional ways of healing most of my life. While studying for my Ayurvedic certification, at times I would pause and think, *Ah, that's what Mumaji was talking about.*

I felt like I was coming full circle, going back to my younger years, then applying this ancient knowledge in a modern setting. My one wish is that I had discovered the connection between Ayurveda and my cherished childhood while

Mumaji was still in this world. I imagine us in her kitchen savouring cups of chai and chatting away as she answered all my questions about things she knew.

Her passing seemed to fire me up to learn more. And as I did, I came to realise that, like my grandmother, I also had a deep interest in the healing power of plants. I have fond memories of us spending hours together in her English garden, especially among the roses and herbs. She always had a tulsi plant (holy basil) in her garden, and now I too keep a tulsi plant on my balcony!

I embarked on a journey of research, delving into the realm of healing botanicals and natural ingredients that could support oral care. Because I'd seen the potential for harm caused by the use of harsh, toxic oral care products throughout my time as a dentist, I was motivated to seek scientific evidence validating the effectiveness of natural ingredients. As a medical professional trained in the Western tradition, I value peer-reviewed and evidence-based scientific research. It is in the meeting of these worlds that we find the perfect union: ancient wisdom supported by cutting-edge research.

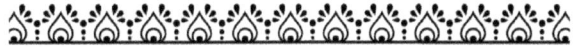

> I embarked on a journey of research, delving into the realm of healing botanicals and natural ingredients that could support oral care.

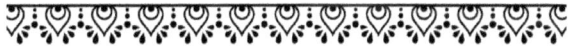

When I realised that very few commercially available products contained these natural, healing ingredients, I decided to apply my knowledge to create something that would go beyond a visit to the dentist. I believe that everyone should have access to oral care products that promote health and wellbeing, free from harmful chemicals. This vision sparked the creation of the Anokhi Veda brand – a comprehensive range of natural Ayurvedic oral care products.

I believe Mumaji's message to me just before she departed was to share with others what I learned from her and from my teachers. To honour her, I decided to write this book – a harmonious blend of her influence, timeless wisdom and my knowledge of modern dentistry – to empower others. *This is what I want to leave behind,* I thought, *a passing on of knowledge that could bene-fit future generations on their way to enhancing their health through dental wellness.*

I offer this book to you, dear reader, in memory of my beloved, late grandmother. It combines my professional experience and my personal journey, blended in a way I hope will demystify any dental concerns you may have and empower you to provide yourself with the best care possible.

May this book serve as a guiding light on your path to achieving optimal oral health.

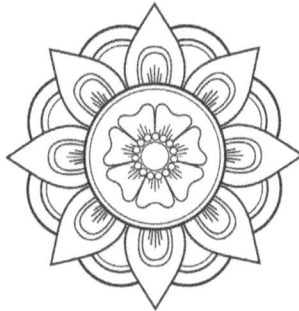

PART 1

Your Mouth Is Your Friend

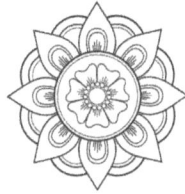

CHAPTER 1

WELCOME TO A NEW WAY OF LOOKING AT YOUR MOUTH

Your Key to Good Health

You want to enjoy good health and live with abundant energy and vitality. You embrace a healthy lifestyle and are mindful of what goes into your body.

You go to yoga class, see a naturopath and visit the chiropractor every now and then. So where does your dental care fit into this conscious way of living?

You may think of your dentist as someone you have to see when a filling falls out or when you are suffering from a toothache. Most of us don't want to go to the dentist. We equate it with pain or, at the very least, some discomfort. Will it hurt? What will my dentist find? Will I lose that tooth that's bothering me?

Or, maybe you see dentistry as a cosmetic service, a way to have a perfect smile with straight, white teeth, just like Hollywood celebrities. But what's going on behind that dazzling smile? Whether we see dentistry as the traditional drill, fill and repair or a beauty-enhancing procedure, we may be missing what our mouths really have to tell us.

Did you know that your mouth is not only the gateway to your gastrointestinal system – your gut – but to your whole body? It holds wisdom and opportunity. By taking care of your mouth, you can enhance so many aspects of your health and even prevent disease. I'm looking forward to showing you how.

3

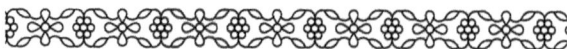

> Whether we see dentistry as the traditional drill, fill and repair or a beauty-enhancing procedure, we may be missing what our mouths really have to tell us.

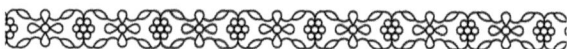

How My Eyes Were Opened

The way I look at patient care and the way I practice dentistry changed on a trip to India a few years after I qualified as a dentist. I remember that day clearly as if it were yesterday.

My family and I were travelling around the deep south of India in the beautiful state of Kerala, home of Ayurveda. Imagine strolling under swaying palm trees or floating along tranquil waterways to small, traditional villages accessible only by houseboat.

As part of our tour, we planned a visit to a spice plantation near the small town where we were staying. Cooking is one of my passions, so I was keen to learn different ways of using the spices and herbs they were growing and hopefully take home some recipes.

I did learn a few new dishes which I still cook to this day. The most memorable part of our tour, though, was when our guide explained in detail how various spices and herbs from plants could be used as medicines for healing. His eyes lit up as he showed us a tulsi plant and told us that crushing the leaves of this sacred Indian herb and breathing in its scent can help a person relax. As I inhaled the sweet fragrance of the leaves, a wave of calm washed over me.

Next, he showed us a moringa plant. Moringa, he said, can strengthen the immune system. I couldn't believe what I was hearing. I'd never thought of plants in this way.

As we walked through the plantation, he explained that in his family's long lineage of practicing Ayurveda, everyday kitchen spices, herbs and even fruits were eaten not only for nourishment but also for their medicinal benefits.

His ancestors didn't have access to doctors with prescription pads and pharmacies, but instead had only the knowledge passed down to them from generations before. This is still the way of medicine in many remote parts of the world, not only in India but also in Africa, South America and other parts of Asia, such as Bali and Thailand.

As I listened, I became more and more interested. It dawned on me that the various herbal concoctions my grandmother had prepared for ailments ranging from coughs and colds to digestive issues were based on the tried-and-true methods of traditional medicine.

That day, a seed was sown. Our tour guide's passion for botanicals ignited my own. When I returned home to Sydney, I wondered about these plants and thought, *if they could be used for health and healing of the body, then surely, couldn't they do the same for the mouth?* And so began my journey into the world of plant medicines and the healing powers of nature for dental health.

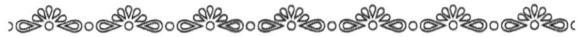

When I returned home to Sydney, I wondered about these plants and thought, *if they could be used for health and healing of the body, then surely, couldn't they do the same for the mouth?*

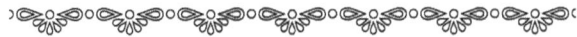

Much to my surprise (and delight), I discovered an abundance of modern research backing up this ancient knowledge. Tulsi, for example, can prevent plaque build-up;[1] cinnamon is highly effective against the decay-causing bacteria S

mutans;[2] and moringa, with its high calcium content, can help remineralise teeth.[3]

The Pharmacy in Your Kitchen

Often without realising it, much of what we need is right under our nose. Imagine: We can build our own dental apothecary from basic spices and herbs in our kitchens, creating remedies and healing for our mouth. Most of the ingredients I am going to tell you about are probably already on your cupboard shelves. For home remedies, we can use those ingredients in multiple ways, from teas to mouthwashes to toothpastes.

The therapeutic effects of plant medicines are often multi-faceted, meaning they have a range of beneficial effects. To name just a few, they can protect us from harmful bacteria and viruses, reduce inflammation and prevent infections, all without the side effects of chemically formulated products.

That's why you may be pleasantly surprised to find that when you choose a botanical to help with dental issues like gum disease or tooth decay, your overall health is enhanced in ways you didn't expect.

Here's an example: As mentioned, in the mouth, tulsi prevents plaque build-up, which can protect against gum disease. In the body, it not only acts as an adaptogen by reducing the effects of stress, but can also lower blood pressure and strengthen the immune system.

Most pharmaceutical drugs, on the other hand, target one specific condition, such as anxiety or high blood pressure, and usually come with a list of undesirable side effects. With botanicals, you receive side *benefits*, not side *effects*.

Care for Your Mouth, Care for Your Body

We are so fortunate to live in times when great advances have been made, not only in the field of medicine but also in dentistry. Throughout nearly three decades of my career, I've witnessed these improvements.

Many of the developments, such as high-speed drills and anaesthetics, mean that dental work today doesn't have to be an unpleasant, painful experience. But these advances have caused us to overlook the bigger picture, which is that our mouths are part of our entire body, not just a home for the teeth and tongue. The mouth and body are in constant communication with

each other, yet modern medicine considers them to be separate from one another.

Our teeth are alive, and they have feelings. I like to think of them as living crystals connected to our vital energy. Tooth decay, gum disease and teeth grinding are not 'normal'. They indicate an imbalance in the body that's asking to be addressed.

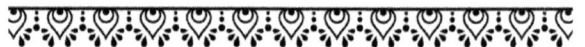

In our modern world, dentists and doctors are educated separately. Dentists focus on the mouth and doctors on the rest of the body. This can make it difficult to view the connection between the two.

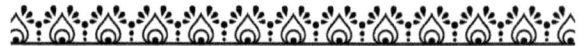

> Tooth decay, gum disease and teeth clenching are not 'normal'. They indicate an imbalance in the body that's asking to be addressed.

It's time to understand that our mouth is integral to our overall health. Let's shift our mindset from 'fix my teeth' to 'help me be healthy and live well'.

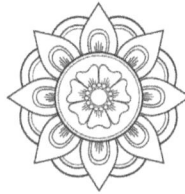

CHAPTER 2

AYURVEDA AND DENTAL HEALTH

How Ancient Wisdom Can Support You

It is 5,000 years ago in ancient India. You rise before the sun, clean your teeth and tongue and swish your mouth with sesame oil. You bathe, pat your skin dry and dress in clean, natural clothing, You continue to embrace the day in this sacred manner by gradually waking up your body, first with deep, rhythmic breathing, then with gentle movements. Meditation anchors your spirit.

You go on to prepare a nourishing breakfast that will sustain you until noon. You eat slowly, mindfully, in preparation for the day ahead.

This is an Ayurveda morning, a day greeted with life-enhancing respect and ritual.

You may think a healing practice that dates back thousands of years and originates in ancient India would have nothing to do with the world of modern dental health. I'm here to tell you otherwise.

During the course of more than twenty-seven years as a dentist, I have unearthed a wealth of knowledge within Ayurveda, much of which I have woven into my own life and the dental care I provide for my patients.

My patients' attitudes toward visiting the dentist, their oral health and their overall wellbeing have all been enhanced as a result of what I've shared with them. Witnessing their transformation has been a rewarding experience for me. I would like to do the same for you.

I'll begin with a brief introduction to Ayurveda – what it is and how it can help you – and show you simple ways you can apply this ancient knowledge in your own life for the wellness you desire.

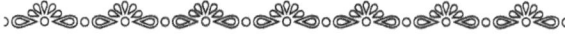

> You may think a healing practice that dates back thousands of years and originates in ancient India would have nothing to do with the world of modern dental health. I'm here to tell you otherwise.

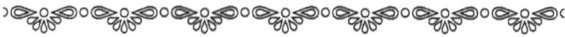

Ayurveda: The Wisdom of Life

First, let me say something about some of the words in this book that may look foreign to you. Ayurveda, because of its antiquity, was originally written in Sanskrit, the language of ancient India. Although it is no longer spoken in modern India, Sanskrit vocabulary has influenced many Indian dialects, just as Latin has influenced modern English and other European languages.

Sanskrit was not only a method of communication, but also served as a foundation for Indian mathematics and science. Because of its logical structure and patterns, the fundamentals of Sanskrit are even being applied to modern-day computer programming, including artificial intelligence – an example of ancient wisdom supporting modern life, just as you will discover in this book.

Because I deeply respect the sacred sound vibration a Sanskrit word carries, on occasion I will use Sanskrit words for certain Ayurvedic terms. Please feel free to skim past them if they feel like too much to take in. As we go along, I'll explain what they mean. Don't worry about the correct pronunciation, and there is certainly no need to learn them by heart.

Here's a start:

The word *Ayurveda* originates in the two Sanskrit words *Ayus*, which means life, and *Veda*, which means wisdom or knowledge. Ayurveda, known as the wisdom of life, is one of the world's oldest holistic healing sciences. More and more people these days look to it as a natural way to care for their health and wellbeing.

I imagine you have come across another word with Sanskrit origins, and that word is *yoga*. Yoga, which means 'union', was originally an ancient spiritual practice. It is now known for its combination of physical postures, breathing and meditation that brings a harmony of body, mind and soul. Yoga has become increasingly popular and is practised by many people all over the planet.[4] You would be hard-pressed not to find a yoga studio or class in almost any corner of the world.

Did you know that yoga and Ayurveda are considered sister sciences? In fact, Ayurveda was a way of life in ancient India long before the practice of yoga became common.

The earliest known references to yoga and Ayurveda appear in the Vedas, the ancient Indian teachings passed down through lineages, initially orally, as many traditions are, and then through written texts.

There is a certain quality to receiving knowledge through spoken words that can't be replicated in written form. To this day, oral teaching remains a tradition in India and other parts of the world.

In Africa, my birthplace, knowledge is traditionally passed down through song and storytelling. This is also the case with the First Nations people of Australia, where I now live. These original custodians of the land have preserved their ancestral knowledge for thousands of years through a form of storytelling and song called the Dreamtime.

I myself have experienced the power of oral teaching. What fond memories I have of learning to cook from my grandmother without any written recipes. She would stand over me at the stove (which at times was quite intimidating!), instructing me how much of each ingredient to put in – a pinch of this, a sprinkle of that, tasting along the way – which gave me the confidence I have in the kitchen today. I can still picture her with one hand on her hip and the other hand pointing out what to do. 'Taste it at this point . . . add this . . . now let it simmer.' Her directions did get me flustered at times, but it was the strict yet loving way she spoke and how she looked that embedded the knowledge deep inside me.

An Eternal Science

Although Ayurveda has been practised for thousands of years, the principles upon which it is based remain the same, which is one of the many reasons I admire it so much. Its science is firmly established and has stood the test of time.

Modern medicine has undoubtedly made many advances over the years, improving the quality of our lives and increasing our lifespans. But we often see conflicting theories, beliefs and practices.

In the pharmaceutical industry, for example, new drugs are formulated and introduced on the market with the aim of treating a specific medical condition, only to be pulled out of circulation once we find they have dangerous side effects that do more harm than good.

As an example, closer to home, within our own kitchens, the debate about whether margarine or butter is better for us has been ongoing for several decades. For centuries, people in many cultures around the world ate butter, recognising its nutritional benefits. In the 1980s, margarine became popular and was suddenly touted as a 'healthier' alternative to butter because of its 'absence of cholesterol'. Butter was considered 'bad' and margarine 'good'. Years later, we know this is not the case.

Margarine is a concoction of chemicals closer to plastic than to real food. The trans fatty acids in margarine are now known to be harmful in multiple ways.[5] They coat our cell walls and increase the chance of heart disease and cancer. Traditional butter, on the other hand, is made from cow's milk. The health benefits of butter and 'good' fats are now widely recognised, and butter has made a comeback as a nutritional food and a staple in our kitchens.

The Ayurvedic version of butter is ghee, a clarified butter made by simmering unsalted butter until the milk solids and the water have separated, leaving behind a golden liquid – ghee – that becomes semi-solid when it cools.

Ghee has always been revered by Indians as a sacred food and consumed for both its nutritional and medicinal benefits, an understanding that hasn't changed over thousands of years.[6]

Holistic Healing Through Ayurveda

Ayurvedic medicine views an individual not as a collection of body parts, such as eyes, teeth, bones and skin, but rather as a whole human being, complete with thoughts, feelings and experiences, as well as a soul.

With all these aspects in mind, the intention of Ayurveda is to maintain a life of balance, health and vitality. 'Health' is not a state defined simply by the results of blood tests, X-rays and scans, but rather as an ongoing and interactive process involving every dimension of life – the physical, the intellectual, the emotional and the spiritual. The true indicator of wellness is the degree to which we have achieved harmony and balance in all of these dimensions.

Ayurveda relies upon three pillars for maintaining that balance: diet *(Aahar)*, sleep *(Nidra)* and the preservation of energy through moderation *(Brahmacharya)*.

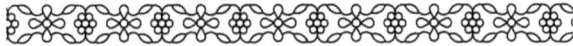

'Health' is not a state defined simply by the results of blood tests, X-rays and scans, but rather as an ongoing and interactive process involving every dimension of life – the physical, the intellectual, the emotional and the spiritual.

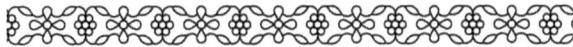

Rather than focus on the treatment of symptoms, Ayurveda's approach is to prevent illness. This is done through practices involving diet and lifestyle, such as yoga, meditation and the use of food as medicine.

When imbalance and disease do occur, Ayurveda seeks to find the underlying contributing factors. What caused the imbalance? To find the root cause, we must lift our sights from just one area of the body and consider the person as the intricate system that they are.

In dentistry too, we are discovering that oral health is much more than we thought it to be. It's not just about teeth and gums. Even stress can affect the mouth, confirming that when we are seeking dental health, we need to consider the person as a whole.[7]

An 'average' person and standardised treatment do not exist in Ayurvedic medicine – yet another example of Ayurveda's holistic nature. Each individual is considered one of a kind, calling for an equally one-of-a-kind plan for maintaining their health. This approach recognises that everyone's expression of health and wellness is their own.

For instance, some of us do better in cold, dry weather, while others are at their best when the climate is warm and humid. You may have a sweet tooth, while your friend favours spicy foods. You may be prone to tooth decay, while someone else struggles with gum disease.

Your needs are unique, and you are your best healer. In this book, you will become an active, empowered participant in your journey toward oral health and wellness. You don't need to attend an Ayurvedic medical school or live in India to understand and apply this knowledge in your daily life. It can be as simple as you like.

One of the fundamentals of holistic healing, whether in Ayurveda or in dentistry, is to seek natural ways to heal ourselves, be it from gum disease or heart disease. With this approach, we can align ourselves with the flow of nature and come back into balance.

Ayurveda offers so many simple ways to enrich wellness by tapping into our body's own wisdom. In the pages ahead, I will share how this knowledge can be used specifically to improve and support our dental health.

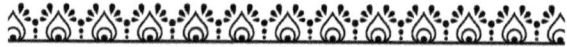

> Ayurveda offers so many simple ways to enrich wellness by tapping into our body's own wisdom.

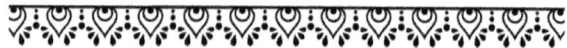

Understanding the Ayurvedic Doshas

According to the principles of Ayurveda, everything in the universe is made up of five fundamental elements: ether (space), air, fire, water and earth.[8]

As humans, we are a microcosm, that is, a small expression of the universe, and so, we too are made up of the same five elements. In Ayurveda these elements are organised into three different energies called 'doshas' referred to as Vata, Pitta and Kapha.

Each of us is made up of all three of these doshas but in different proportions that are uniquely our own. Usually, the energies of one or two doshas stand out more than the others. One person may primarily exhibit Vata traits, while another may carry more Kapha qualities. In Ayurvedic medicine, a person's physical, mental and emotional health is determined by their dosha make-up, the genetic blueprint they were born with, called *Prakruti* in Ayurveda.

In the dosha descriptions that follow, I've provided both general characteristics and those I see in my dental patients. Look over these descriptions and see which ones resonate with you. To find out your own Prakruti, you can complete the Ayurveda Dosha Quiz in Appendix A.

Vata Dosha

The elements that make up Vata dosha are air and empty space (also known as ether). If you are predominantly Vata in energy, you are likely to have a slim build; long, slender limbs; dry skin; and a tendency to lose weight. You are highly active, but your energy can be easily depleted.

Vata-dominant people tend to be sensitive to cold, dry weather and prefer locations that are warmer and more humid. When they are out of balance, they're likely to experience gut issues such as bloating and constipation due to the dry, airy nature of their dosha. They may also have bad breath. Vata individuals tend to be sensitive to stress and can frequently suffer from anxiety even though they are naturally creative, spontaneous and impulsive. Many artists and performers are dominated by Vata dosha, which is the energy of movement and change. If we were to look at the animal kingdom, I would say the characteristics of a sparrow best exemplify Vata.

During my work as a dentist, I have noticed that Vata-dominant patients usually have porous, sensitive teeth and may experience issues like dental crowding inside their small, narrow jaws. Their lips are often dry and cracked, and their gums may be thin, dark and receding. They may experience dental anxiety and can take longer to recover from dental treatment than my patients who are predominantly Pitta or Kapha.

Pitta Dosha

Pitta dosha is made up of the elements of fire and water. If you are predominately Pitta in nature, you have a medium build and can keep your weight stable. You tend to have a strong appetite and good digestion. You may have a low tolerance for heat and a tendency to get sunburned; hence, you prefer cooler environments. When you are out of balance, you are likely to get overheated.

Pitta-dominant people have perceptive and analytical minds and are quite often hardworking and meticulous. They are goal-oriented and enjoy planning and being organised. Although they are good at managing their energy, they can become easily frustrated and angry and have a tendency for burnout. The energy of many CEOs and highly driven achievers tends to be dominated by Pitta. An example of Pitta energy in the animal world is that of a lion.

My patients whose primary dosha is Pitta typically have plump, tender gums and red, moist lips. Their teeth are usually moderate in size and properly aligned. Because an imbalance in Pitta energy can cause inflammation, these patients often suffer from cold sores and bleeding gums. They are very structured in their approach to dental care. They want to know what they should do, when and for how long.

Kapha Dosha

Earth and water are the elements that make up Kapha dosha. If you are predominately Kapha in nature, you likely have a stocky build and tend to be on the heavier side. Your skin tone is close to olive, you may prefer warm, dry climates and be sensitive to high levels of humidity.

Even though they are naturally laid back and relaxed, when Kapha-dominant people are out of balance, they can become stuck in a rut and feel unmotivated. They are prone to lethargic and depressive states and may have to push themselves to get out and exercise. Kapha types are well suited to administrative or caregiving positions that require a patient, long-term view, such as teaching, childcare and nursing. This is because Kapha individuals are renowned for being reliable and steady. In the animal kingdom, the energy of an elephant best describes Kapha dosha because of its heavy, slow-moving nature.

In my dental practice, I have noticed that patients who are predominantly Kapha tend to have strong, pearly-white teeth that are resistant to decay, thick lips and a large tongue. They may suffer from an imbalance in the pH level of their mouths, which can lead to an overgrowth of yeast, often seen as a white coating on the tongue. They may also experience imbalances in saliva production, which can present as either a dry mouth or excessive salivation. My Kapha patients might be slow to pick up new dental care habits, but once they do, they continue in a committed and steady manner.

Balancing the Doshas

From what you've learned about Ayurveda so far, you know that disease occurs when we lose our internal equilibrium.

Here are three ways you can help yourself return to a state of balance:

- Balance the energy of the dosha that is out of balance.
- Balance your energies with the three pillars of Ayurveda.
- Examine your relationship with your external environment.

Because Ayurveda focuses on an individual's unique needs, we can consider ways to balance our particular dosha. In general, that involves giving our senses the opposite experience of the dosha quality that has fallen out of alignment. In other words, if we've become overweight, we need to eat more lightly. To calm our racing minds, we can turn to meditation or reconnect with nature for grounding.

As someone whose predominant dosha is Vata, I tend to feel chilly, have dry skin and can easily deplete my energy levels. So, whenever I feel off-kilter, the support I require consists of applying the opposite qualities: warmth, moisture and rest. I take self-care measures such as drinking ginger tea, massaging my body with warming sesame oil and prioritising an early bedtime.

My grandmother, on the other hand, was a Pitta-dominant person. When I was young, I would watch as she massaged her head with coconut oil, which is cooling in nature, and then leave it in her hair overnight. She did this every night. In hindsight, I realise she was trying to alleviate the heat of Pitta dosha. She also liked to add mint leaves to her morning chai because mint has a naturally cooling effect on the body.

In Ayurvedic medicine, restoring our balance and health no matter what our dosha make-up requires us to examine our diet, our sleep and our energy expenditure, the three pillars I talked about earlier.

Sometimes all it takes is a small tweak to what we've been doing – adding an avocado to our daily menu, going to bed fifteen minutes earlier or consciously avoiding distressing newscasts.

This brings me to an important Ayurvedic principle: How we live with our external world affects our internal world. And it's what goes on inside us that forms the essence of our health, our *Ojas*, the Sanskrit word for vitality.

Picture yourself basking in the comforting warmth of sunlight, absorbing the sun's healing rays. For most of us, even the Pitta-dominant, some amount of sunshine feels good. It's certainly true for me. After even twenty minutes in the sun, I feel revitalised.

Modern research confirms the importance of sunlight for our wellbeing.[9] The sun's rays play an important role in stimulating our bodies to make vitamin D, a vital nutrient that supports our immune system and various internal processes. And when sunlight is absorbed through our eyes, it activates the pineal gland to make melatonin, a hormone essential for sleep.

By consciously aligning our external choices with our inner nature, we can cultivate a life of harmony and balance. Whether it involves understanding and addressing our specific dosha needs, evaluating our diet, sleep patterns and energy expenditure or exploring new ways to interact with the world around us, Ayurveda can show us the way.

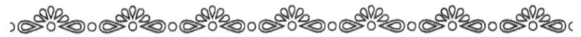

> By consciously aligning our external choices with our inner nature, we can cultivate a life of harmony and balance.

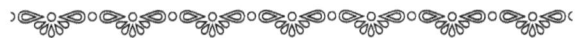

Three Ways Ayurveda Can Support Our Dental Health

While writing this book, my family and friends would ask me what Ayurveda had to do with dentistry. 'Quite a lot!' I would say. Ayurveda holds much wisdom on how to maintain good oral health by acknowledging the intricate connections between our mouth, digestive system and overall vitality.

Here are three key areas of Ayurvedic wisdom that have enriched how I care for my patients:

- Establish a daily oral care routine.
- Use plant-based remedies to support the oral microbiome.
- Understand that the health of our gut affects our mouth and vice versa.

Let me explain.

Dinacharya: A Daily Routine for Balance Throughout the Day

If we look at the natural world around us, we will see rhythms and cycles everywhere. The sun rises and sets each day at predictable times, the moon waxes and wanes every month and the seasons come and go throughout the year.

As human beings, we, too, live by cycles. Sometimes our immune system is strong and at other times it's vulnerable. Women have menstrual cycles, and men also experience hormonal fluctuations. Within a given day, our circadian rhythms control when we feel hungry and when we feel sleepy, when we have energy and when we are tired.

If we, as a part of nature, tune ourselves to the rhythms and cycles of the natural world, we will experience grounding, clarity and vitality. These qualities help us build resilience in dealing with our fast-paced modern world, where speed, noise and constant change can be unsettling.

Would you like to learn how to tune yourself to nature's rhythms so that you too can experience a state of ease and wellbeing? Ayurveda has a way. It's called *Dinacharya*, which means 'to follow the knowledge of the day'. The story I told you at the beginning of this chapter was an example of greeting the day with gratitude and respect in alignment with nature that can bring you deep benefits.

Looking back, I realise that my grandmother followed a *Dinacharya* through her morning routine and other activities throughout the day. She had a night-time routine as well, called *Ratricharya* in Ayurveda. (*Dina* means day and *Ratri*, night. *Acharya* means activity.)

Even the world of business recognises the importance of a daily routine for professional success.[10] With Ayurveda, you can establish a daily routine that will serve as a foundation for success in all aspects of your health and wellbeing.

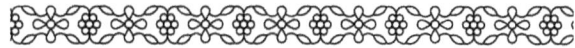

What does it mean to 'follow the knowledge of the day'? Quite simply, it refers to the practice of carrying out our daily actions at specific times so that they flow with nature's rhythms – when we should eat, for example, when we should be active and when we should sleep.

And because Ayurveda has always recognised that good oral health is essential for whole body health, it places great emphasis on including dental hygiene in our daily routine. Later, I'll walk you through step by step in designing your very own 'Oral Dinacharya'. You'll be able to create a quick and simple oral care routine based on your specific needs.

Our mouths do need special care. Of course, you recognise the mouth as vital for eating, drinking and talking. You may not realise, however, that there is a great deal more activity going on in there.

Not only does the mouth have a rich blood and nerve supply, but it also has its very own diverse ecosystem of bacteria and other microorganisms known as the oral microbiome.

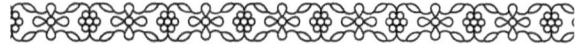

> With Ayurveda, you can establish a daily routine that will serve as a foundation for success in all aspects of your health and wellbeing.

It is estimated that a typical adult's mouth is home to anywhere between fifty and one hundred billion bacteria.[11] Some are helpful, and some are harmful. It's like an entire universe living inside your mouth.

The oral microbiome is a relatively new, yet rapidly growing area of study. I'm delighted because I believe it is key to our future understanding (and prevention) of dental (and systemic) disease. It deserves its place right up there with the gut microbiome.

Within the oral microbiome, there are different ecosystems just as there are different suburbs within a city. One lies on the surface of the tongue, another in the gum pockets, one on the teeth and yet another in dental plaque. Different types of bacteria live in each ecosystem.[12]

When we look at a healthy mouth on a microscopic level, the bacteria are in balance and are able to live quite happily with each other. Helpful bacteria keep our mouths and us healthy, and they keep the harmful bacteria in check.

When the environment of the mouth or body is unhealthy, however, it can lead to acidity, which creates an opportunity for harmful bacteria to proliferate and take over.

Consider the Amazon rainforest as one example of a particular type of ecosystem. If the environment is kept healthy and free of pollutants, the plants and animals all flourish and thrive as intended by nature.

If the harmful bacteria in our mouth are swallowed or absorbed into our bloodstream, they can travel to other parts of the digestive system and body and trigger inflammation in sites like the stomach, colon, brain, joints and heart. For this reason, we need to respect and look after the vital ecosystem that is our oral microbiome.

One way we can do this is by being careful not to use toothpastes and mouthwashes containing harsh, toxic chemicals.[13] These ingredients wipe out all the bacteria indiscriminately, just as deforestation strips the land and air of the elements we need.[14]

Instead, why not look to what nature has provided us for healing: herbs, spices and plant medicines that can help bring our body and oral microbiome into balance.

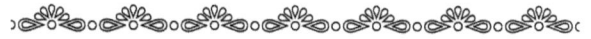

> If the harmful bacteria in our mouth are swallowed or absorbed into our bloodstream, they can travel to other parts of the digestive system and body and trigger inflammation in sites like the stomach, colon, brain, joints and heart.

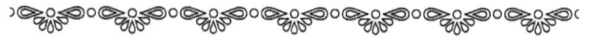

Calling on Plant Medicines to Keep the Mouth Healthy

Ayurveda has long acknowledged the healing potential of plant medicines, both for oral health and for the treatment of diseases affecting the whole body. The benefits these herbs and spices offer to the mouth are just now starting to be confirmed by modern research as you will see in the studies cited throughout this book.

Even if manufacturers are slow to include natural ingredients in their products, there is nothing stopping you from incorporating them into your personal oral hygiene practice.

The beauty of natural ingredients like herbs and spices is that they have an innate intelligence and know exactly what to do once inside our bodies. They draw to themselves the harmful bacteria, viruses and fungi that should not be living in the body and destroy them, whilst leaving the beneficial ones alone. We want helpful bacteria in our mouth and gut. Botanicals leave them there.

You can enjoy the benefits of a healthy mouth and support your body's health by brushing your teeth and rinsing your mouth with products containing natural spices, herbs, minerals and clays. These ingredients can give you a fresh, clean mouth without causing harm to your body.

Let's give the oral microbiome and the mouth the attention and respect they deserve – on par with the gut. Think about it. The mouth is where digestion begins. Make sure you give your digestion the best possible start by caring for your mouth. Then, enhance your oral health even more by looking to Ayurvedic wisdom to support your entire digestive system.

Agni: Supporting the Mouth–Gut Connection

Ayurvedic medicine has always placed great emphasis on the importance of digestive health. These days, the health and wellness industry is abuzz with terms like 'gut health', 'microbiome' and 'probiotics' as more and more modern studies validate what has always been known to be true in Ayurveda.[15]

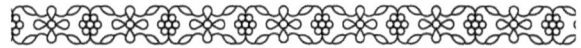

> Let's give the oral microbiome and the mouth the attention and respect they deserve – on par with the gut.

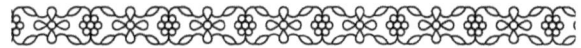

We've come to understand that the bacteria that live in our gut have an effect on nearly every part of our body. Take our immune system, for example. We now know that over seventy per cent of our immune cells reside in the digestive system rather than in the blood.[16] This means the health of our immunity and our digestive system are closely intertwined. And because the mouth is part of the digestive system, it plays an important role in our immune health.

In Ayurveda, the strength of our digestive system is referred to as our 'digestive fire' and is called *Agni*, the Sanskrit word for fire.[17] Although not a literal fire, our digestive Agni is a representation of the element of fire, which is responsible for transforming the food we eat into energy.

Ayurveda's understanding of Agni includes the gut microbiome, even if ancient texts did not use the word 'microbiome'. Agni encompasses all the activities modern medicine views as contributors to the metabolic process of breaking down food and absorbing the nutrients it contains: the enzymes in our mouth and those secreted by our stomach and pancreas, the bile from our liver and the hydrochloric acid in our stomach.

When Agni is weak, meaning our digestive system isn't working well, we can experience an accumulation of toxins in the body, which can in turn open the door to many diseases. By 'toxin', I mean any harmful substance that is made either externally in the world around us (bacteria, viruses, environmental contaminants, heavy metals) or internally by our own body (carbon dioxide, ammonia, lactic acid, free radicals). In Ayurveda, undigested food and other toxins in the body are called *Ama,* which I will talk about more later in this chapter.

From an Ayurvedic perspective, it is believed that the root cause of most disease can be traced to a problem in the gut, which is something I have personally witnessed throughout my work over the years.

Although the cause and symptoms of a digestive issue can differ from person to person, one thing appears to be consistent across the board: Maintaining a healthy gut is vital to maintaining a healthy body.[18] Poor digestion is one of the main reasons people gain weight, have low energy levels, develop brain fog, experience accelerated ageing and suffer from a variety of ailments.[19]

In my dental practice, particularly in recent years, I've seen a dramatic increase in digestive health issues such as reflux, leaky gut syndrome, irritable bowel syndrome (IBS) and small intestinal bacterial overgrowth (SIBO). Some of these disorders I'd never heard of when I was training to be a dentist thirty years ago.

My patients are frequently taken aback when I inquire about their toilet habits. They are curious as to why a dentist would ask such a question. I ask because gut health affects oral health and oral health affects gut health. The digestive tract is a single organ, one tube, much like a garden hose, with the mouth as the first part of that hose. When one part is unhealthy, the health of the whole system suffers.

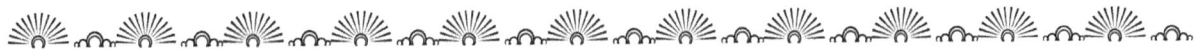

CRIME AGAINST WISDOM

In today's world, we have the luxury of being able to consume anything we want, whenever we want, regardless of the time of year. This may be viewed as one of the great advances of the modern world; however, this so-called 'advancement' can lead us to ignore our body's innate wisdom.

When we step away from the true purpose of eating and drinking, which is to nourish ourselves on a mind–body–spirit level, we forget to eat in alignment with our body's true needs.

Our bodies are incredibly intelligent and can speak to us through our intuition, telling us what we need to nourish ourselves. Imagine the comfort of drinking a bowl of hot soup on a cold winter's day or a plate of watermelon on a hot summer's day. We instinctively know what to eat throughout the seasons to provide us with what we need.

When we choose to reject this knowledge by eating a large meal just before bed or eating chilled watermelon on a cold day, which adds cold to cold, we are ignoring what our bodies truly need. Ayurveda refers to this as *Prajnaparadha*, which literally translates to 'a crime against wisdom'.

In the Ayurvedic tradition, it is believed that the majority of illness and disease arises because we make poor lifestyle choices, all the while knowing they are not wise ones. Think about it for yourself, how good you feel after eating a fresh, nourishing meal as opposed to processed junk food.

Sometimes all that's required of us to make decisions that support our wellbeing is to trust our gut feelings. Our bodies are wise.

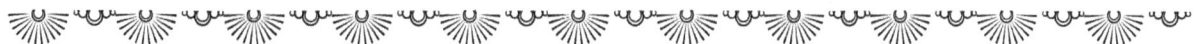

If we have poor gut health (in other words, weak Agni), a number of problems can arise in the mouth.

Consider a common disorder known as acid reflux in which the acidic contents of the stomach flow back up the esophagus into the throat, where it may expose the teeth to acid. That acid can cause the surface minerals of the teeth to disintegrate, leading to tooth erosion[20] and sensitivity. Reflux can also make the environment of the mouth more acidic, shifting the balance of the oral microbiome from a healthy one to a more disease-like state where cavities and gum disease may develop.[21]

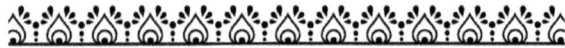

> The digestive tract is a single organ, one tube, much like a garden hose, with the mouth as the first part of that hose.

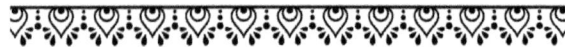

Even bad breath can be the result of digestive issues. Many of my patients who suffer from halitosis have underlying digestive problems such as acid reflux or chronic constipation. While swishing with chemical-based mouthwashes, sucking on mints and even daily tongue scraping may offer temporary relief, the issue of bad breath will persist as long as the digestive issue remains.

Painful mouth ulcers can also arise from digestive problems such as malabsorption (which results in nutritional deficiencies in B vitamins, iron and other minerals) and inflammatory diseases of the gut like Crohn's disease and ulcerative colitis.[22]

In turn, problems in our mouth can affect our gut. If you're missing teeth, you might not be able to chew your food thoroughly. The mouth is where the digestion of carbohydrates and fats should begin.[23] If it doesn't happen there, the food particles are passed in their partially digested state to the small intestine, where it will be difficult to absorb the nutrients contained in the food. So, no matter how good the quality of food you're eating, if it's not being digested and absorbed, it's of no use.

Recall how I talked earlier about Ama, the Ayurvedic term for undigested food and other toxins. Think of Ama as a thick, sticky substance produced internally from stagnating, unmetabolised food. It clogs our body's natural processes and prevents them from working as they should.[24]

Ama in the mouth – toxins created by oral infections, for example – can also have an effect on the gut microbiome. We usually end up swallowing those toxins if the infection is left untreated. It has recently come to light that certain types of stomach and bowel cancers may be caused by harmful bacteria originating in the mouth.[25]

In a similar vein, if you have a dry mouth because of medications you take or because you breathe through your mouth, you'll have less saliva. Saliva contains our digestive enzymes. Without these essential enzymes, your food won't be broken down as it should be and will create Ama.

Do you see the reciprocal relationship between dental health and gut health?

Ayurveda offers us general guidelines for strengthening our Agni as well as dietary recommendations tailored to our specific dosha make-up. There's a vast amount of information in books and on the internet offering dietary guidelines from an Ayurvedic perspective. I've offered a few of these resources in Appendix B.

We can tap into Ayurvedic wisdom and incorporate simple recommendations into our daily lives that will keep our digestive health – our Agni – strong.

When I was learning about Ayurveda, I pictured Agni as a pot of simmering water on a stovetop. We must keep that pot warm so the water inside can process any food we add to it, just as our inner Agni needs to be kept warm so that we can easily and efficiently digest our food.

Below are some simple tips I give my patients to keep the pot on the stove warm and the fire of Agni kindled. I invite you to choose one to incorporate into your life now and then add others gradually. Each will serve you well.

Simple Ways to Strengthen Your Agni

- Align your eating habits with the natural cycles of the day. What exactly does this mean? According to Ayurveda, the power of Agni (our digestive fire) fluctuates in the same way as the sun, which represents our universal fire. The sun's rays are at their most powerful when they're directly above us in the middle of the day. The same is true of our Agni.

  For this reason, Ayurveda suggests that lunch be the largest meal of the day and be eaten as close to midday as possible. The second-heaviest meal should be breakfast, consumed no later than eight in the morning. That makes dinner our lightest meal of the day. It should be eaten at least two to three hours before going to bed so our digestive organs have time to rest and repair while we sleep.

It's easy to see how our customary, modern way of living differs from the philosophy of Ayurveda. Skipping breakfast and eating a large meal late at night can contribute to poor digestive health.

- Notice how you're taking in beverages. Avoid cold, iced drinks and refrain from gulping down whatever it is you're drinking. As most of our immune system is located throughout our digestive tract, including the throat and tonsils, we don't want to weaken our immunity by dampening it with cold drinks. Imagine adding ice water to that simmering pot of water you have on the stove.

When we experience a sore throat, a cold or the flu, our bodies instinctively guide us to take in warm drinks. Again, notice how different this is from our contemporary way of living. We are accustomed to drinking cold drinks, and the majority of restaurants serve beverages with ice cubes. It's time to reconsider this habit.

- Eat in harmony with the seasons and shop locally for fresh produce. Let nature design your menu. Your plate should be composed of vegetables, fruits and nutrient-dense foods, including protein and healthy fats such as those found in ghee, avocados, nuts and seeds.

The universality of Ayurveda's basic principles make them applicable regardless of the dietary pattern you've chosen due to health concerns, ethical considerations or religious beliefs.

- Activate your digestive process well before the food reaches your lips. How? Listen to your food being cooked. The sounds of sizzling and boiling can make you hungry and stimulate your digestive processes. The same activation can take place when we look at images of food.

Get messy and eat with your hands. According to Ayurveda, when we touch food, it stimulates our digestion by alerting our stomach to what it will soon be receiving. Throughout history, people have used their hands to eat. In remote parts of the world, they still do. It's only recently that cutlery has developed into its modern form. Before I started going to school, I spent my childhood eating with my hands, as has been the custom in India since ancient times. This is how everyone in my family ate, and I finally understand the reasoning behind it.

- Check your emotions. Always be mindful of your emotional state while you're cooking. My grandmother used to advise me against preparing or consuming food when feeling upset, as she believed that negative energy could be absorbed into the food.

- Eat with a Mindful, not a Mind Full, presence.[26] Once your food is prepared, savour it in a peaceful environment. Let it nourish both your body and soul. Eat mindfully, avoid distractions from technology, and allow yourself to fully appreciate and engage with the nourishment before you.

When I was a child, my parents had a rule that we all had to sit together as a family at the dining table for dinner, without the television or other distractions. It was a peaceful time for us to come together and connect at the end of the day. During my school years, many of my friends were allowed to watch TV while eating with trays on their laps, referred to back then as TV dinners. At the time, I felt envious and resented my parents for not allowing me to do the same. As I've grown older, however, I've come to understand and appreciate their perspective and have adopted it for myself.

- Make a habit of chewing each mouthful at least twenty-five times. This helps break down the food into smaller particles that can be further digested in the stomach and intestines. As the saying goes, 'Chew your liquids and drink your foods.'

- Eat until you just begin to feel full, which corresponds to roughly eighty per cent of your stomach's capacity. This leaves the remaining twenty per cent as space for the food to mix thoroughly with your digestive juices. You are allowing Agni to do its job.

Now that you have learned how Ayurveda connects to oral health and understand my approach to dentistry, join me to see how it all comes together in practice with my patients.

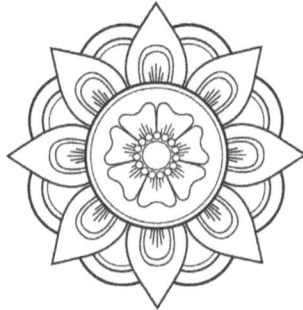

PART 2

What Is Your Mouth Telling You?

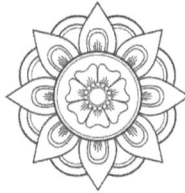

CHAPTER 3

GUM DISEASE

The King of Deception

Julian hadn't been to the dentist often, perhaps just four or five times in his sixty-four years. His approach to life and to his health, was, 'If it ain't broke, why fix it?'

He had booked an appointment with me because over the past couple of months, he'd noticed one of his lower molars had become loose. And in recent weeks, the tooth had become tender and sore when chewing even soft foods.

'I saw a dentist a few years ago,' he told me, 'just for a cleaning and some teeth whitening. My daughter was getting married, and I wanted to look good in the wedding photos. The dentist mentioned something about my needing to come back for a proper check-up, but time just got away from me.'

And time did get away from Julian. He was a busy corporate lawyer working long hours with very little time for self-care. Unfortunately, a year ago, he suffered a heart attack, which necessitated surgery and prompted him to retire.

'Tell me about your heart attack,' I said.

'It rattled me, that's for sure. I didn't know what was happening or if I would make it. I ended up having two stents put in. Now I have to take blood thinners every day.'

'At least since I've retired, I'm under less stress and can focus on getting healthier. I've started a few exercises my cardiologist suggested, and I'm going for a long walk every morning.' His face softened, and I sensed his pride in the changes he'd made.

As I looked at the new patient form he had completed, I saw Julian was also taking medications for high cholesterol and a stomach ulcer.

'It's been a rough couple of years,' he said. 'Most of my life I've been so healthy.'

'That must be hard for you,' I said. 'Before I look in your mouth, I have a couple more questions. Can you tell me about your oral care routine? How do you look after your teeth and gums?'

'I brush my teeth every night,' he said, 'and swish with a mouthwash my wife buys from the supermarket. She's always complaining I have bad breath.' He half-laughed, but I could tell it embarrassed him.

'Do you ever brush in the morning or clean your tongue?' I asked.

'Clean my tongue? I've never heard of that.'

'Okay,' I said, 'we'll go over that later. And your gums? Do they feel healthy to you?'

'They seem okay except around that loose tooth. The gum there feels sore. My gums do bleed a little when I brush, but they feel fine.'

I knew that bleeding gums were not 'fine'. Even a small amount of bleeding suggests something is not right and that the body is sending blood, which contains our immune cells, to help protect the affected area. I say to my patients, 'Pink in the sink is not okay.' If our eyes bled every day when we washed our face, we would be concerned. We should be just as concerned about bleeding gums.

When I looked inside Julian's mouth, I immediately saw that his gums were red and puffy instead of pink and firm. This is known as *gingivitis* (inflammation of the gums).

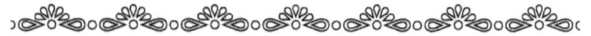

> I say to my patients, 'Pink in the sink is not okay.' If our eyes bled every day when we washed our face, we would be concerned.

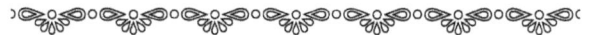

His gums were also loose around his teeth, much like a polo-neck jumper that has lost snugness around the neck. This loosening was forming space between his teeth and gums, what we call pockets, which I measured with a dental probe.

I placed the probe into each of Julian's gum pockets. How far the probe went down would tell me, in millimetres, how serious Julian's gingivitis was.

Healthy gum pockets are 1–2 mm deep. If my probe measures a depth of 4 mm or more, advanced gum disease has set in. Most of Julian's pockets measured between 3 and 4 mm, which indicates moderate gum disease, but the pocket around the loose tooth measured 9 mm. And all of his gums bled as soon as I probed them. This was not a good sign.

Our gum pockets have low levels of oxygen. Harmful bacteria in the mouth tend to be anaerobic, meaning they prefer to live where there is little to no oxygen. This means these pockets become the perfect little luxury resorts in which to take up residence.

'Julian,' I said, 'it looks like you have a problem here. The tooth itself is sound, but the gum around it doesn't look healthy.'

When his eyes met mine, I saw his concern.

Julian's puffy, bleeding gums and deep gum pockets, along with his bad breath, were all classic signs of periodontitis, also referred to as gum disease.

'This is called periodontal disease, Julian. It's actually a common, and unfortunately, often undetected problem. It affects three in ten adult Australians. That's almost a third of the adults in this country.'[27]

I hoped it reassured Julian to know he wasn't alone.

'Let's take an X-ray. The gum inflammation I can see may be affecting the bone that supports and anchors the teeth. An X-ray will help us look deeper.'

X-rays are a helpful diagnostic tool in the field of dentistry. When a dentist looks in your mouth, they can see only one-third of the full picture. They can't see between the teeth, which is a common site for decay, nor view the nearly two-thirds of teeth submerged in bone. X-rays are also helpful to dentists in assessing the jawbones for bone levels, infections, cysts and other hidden activity.

Julian was fine about having X-rays, but in my practice, not all patients are. Although newer technology in dentistry exposes us to much lower levels of radiation than traditional X-ray machines, many people are still anxious about the procedure.

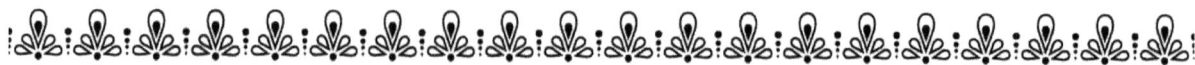

DEMYSTIFYING THE TERMINOLOGY

It's easy to get lost in all the professional jargon. Both gingivitis and periodontitis are within a spectrum of the same disease.

Gingivitis is inflammation of the gums.

Periodontitis, or periodontal disease, is inflammation of both the gums and the bone supporting the teeth, although it is often referred to as 'gum disease'.

Most people experience gingivitis at some point in their lives. I've seen it in patients who have been slack with their oral care or have been through a period of acute stress, illness or demand, such

as pregnancy, which has depleted their energy, nutritional state or immunity. This inflammation can usually be resolved with good oral care and efforts to restore overall health.

The mild symptoms of gingivitis can make it easy to ignore, but if it persists and is not treated, it may turn into a bigger problem. Gingivitis doesn't always lead to periodontitis, but periodontitis is usually preceded by gingivitis.

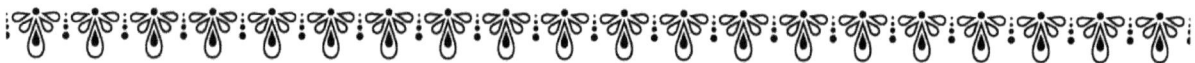

Natural Protection Against Radiation

To protect against the potential effects of radiation, certain Ayurvedic spices can be beneficial. These include clove,[28] cinnamon,[29] ginger[30] and turmeric,[31] which are known for their antioxidant properties that can help neutralise free radicals and reduce oxidative stress in the body.

You can prepare a simple herbal tea by steeping these ingredients in hot water and sipping the infusion before and after your dental appointment. Or, you can add the spices to a traditional chai recipe (black tea infused with spices and milk) or prepare Golden Milk, a soothing Ayurvedic drink made with turmeric, warm milk and other spices.

Antioxidant-rich teas like tulsi,[32] triphala[33] or mint[34] can also help offset the effects of radiation.[35]

For Julian, we took a reduced radiation orthopantomogram (OPG) X-ray, which gives a panoramic view of all the bones and teeth in one image. The OPG showed Julian had lost a lot of bone around his teeth, and hardly any bone remained around the sore tooth he was complaining of. No wonder it was loose.

Now we were talking about something beyond gingivitis. Because Julian's underlying bone was involved, dissolving away and reducing anchorage for his teeth, we had entered the territory known as periodontal disease or periodontitis.

Gum Disease, the Silent House Guest

'I just don't understand,' Julian said. 'I've never had any problems with my teeth before now. How can I suddenly have this thing you call periodontal disease?'

He'd had enough medical surprises in the past two years. I'm sure he didn't need more. I went on to explain.

'Periodontal disease doesn't necessarily cause pain or problems in its early stages. It's only when it reaches a more advanced state that other symptoms appear, like bad breath, loose teeth and pain. You may not have realised it, but this condition has likely been progressing for years. It's tied to the health of the plaque in your mouth. And the health of your body.'

Plaque (also called biofilm) is that sticky film you feel when you run your tongue over your teeth. It's made up of food particles, saliva and microbiome bacteria.

When plaque mixes with minerals in the saliva, it becomes calculus, also known as tartar, a harder build-up on the teeth that can't be removed by just brushing and flossing. It's like the scale of mineral deposit that forms at the bottom of a kettle and is most likely what Julian's dentist cleaned off his teeth before his daughter's wedding.

'Would you like to see the plaque on your teeth?' I asked Julian.

'Yes, please.'

I gave Julian a disclosing tablet which is made up of a bright pink vegetable dye that sticks to soft dental plaque and stains it. I asked him to chew on the tablet and then rinse his mouth. When he was done, I handed him a mirror.

'Whatever looks pink on your teeth is plaque.'

'That's a lot of pink,' he said. 'Is that bad?'

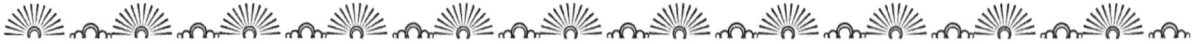

YOUR TONGUE: NATURE'S BEST DENTAL TOOL

Did you know that the tongue is covered in millions of nerve endings? This makes it a highly sensitive organ for perception.

Perhaps you've noticed when eating that if there is the slightest bit of grit in your food or a tiny piece of packaging, your tongue will be sure to find it. If that same piece fell, say, on top of your foot, you may not even feel it.

Because our mouth is the gateway to the body, we need our tongue to be this 'bouncer' at the door.

Use your tongue to feel around your mouth. Can you feel the sticky plaque? Is there food stuck between or on your teeth?

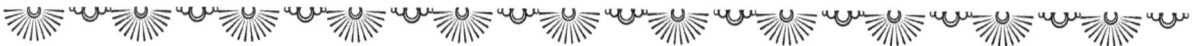

'Well, yes and no,' I replied. 'Healthy plaque is important for the health of our mouth. We actually need it.'

'Really?'

'First of all, it can help strengthen our teeth by encouraging minerals in the saliva to coat and protect the teeth.

'Second, when we look at plaque from a healthy mouth under a microscope, we can see it's made up of mainly aerobic bacteria, bacteria that thrive in an oxygen-rich environment. These are the helpful bacteria, the ones we want lots of.

They keep our mouth healthy by making hydrogen peroxide, a natural disinfectant, which releases oxygen and destroys the harmful, anaerobic bacteria, keeping their numbers in check.[36]

'Those helpful bacteria also make nitric oxide, an important messenger to the muscles surrounding our blood vessels, telling them to relax, which helps lower our blood pressure.

'When our plaque has an abundance of helpful bacteria, our teeth feel clean, our gums look pink and don't bleed and our breath is fresh.'

Julian nodded.

'Dental plaque has been in mouths for thousands of years,' I told him. 'Researchers have studied the fossilised plaque in Neanderthal skulls, and what they've discovered is interesting.[37]

'They found lots of plaque and tartar build-up on their teeth but not the level of dental disease we experience in today's world. That's because their dental plaque was somewhat healthier than ours, even without fancy toothbrushes, toothpastes or professional cleans.'

'How could that be?' Julian said.

'I believe it comes down to their diet and how they lived – so different from how we eat and live these days. As we've evolved, our oral microbiome has changed and become less healthy.'

If we look back in time, our oral microbiome underwent significant changes following two big shifts in our evolutionary history: The first major event, around 10,000 years ago, was the transition from a lifestyle of hunting and gathering to agriculture and farming, which meant we began to eat more carbohydrate-rich foods. As a result, the oral microbiome became more populated with harmful bacteria, the bacteria responsible for problems such as bad breath, bleeding gums and dental decay.

The biggest change in the health of our mouth, however, came with the Industrial Revolution in the 18th century, when it became easy to process and package food with machines. By the late 1800s, we were beginning to eat a more modernised diet consisting of white flour, sugar and processed foods.[38] This led to even more changes in our oral microbiome, which became less diverse in bacteria – not a good thing. We need a variety of microorganisms for our immunity and our health.

Eating softer foods meant less chewing, and our jaw muscles didn't have to work as hard when we ate. Those muscles got smaller and smaller as we evolved, as did our jaws, in part to accommodate our growing brains. As a result, our teeth are now often crowded and misaligned, with little or no room for wisdom teeth.

Alongside shrinking jaws, our nasal passages narrowed to make room for a larger brain, which led to compromised breathing. Many of us now breathe through our mouth instead of our nose. Mouth breathing can cause many problems, from dry mouth to sleep deprivation to anxiety.[39]

Our ancestors' jaws, in contrast, were wide and strong, and their nasal passages were spacious and well developed. If you search online for hunter-gatherer skull images, you'll see for yourself the difference in human skulls between now and then.

As the industrial era progressed, we abandoned the primitive wisdom practice of living according to the laws of nature in which we ate seasonally appropriate, nutrient-dense foods. You'll learn more about the consequences of this shift away from a natural diet in the next chapter on tooth decay.

At the same time, we've seen a sharp rise globally in allergies and degenerative diseases such as diabetes, cancer and autoimmune disorders. Most of them are inflammatory in nature, just like gum disease.

The decline in our health mirrors the decline in the health of our planet. In the past one hundred years our planet has become sicker, and so have we.

Because of the change in what we eat and how we live, our mouths and bodies have become more acidic.[40] Acidity sets the stage for disease, while alkalinity supports health, including the health of the plaque sitting around our teeth. Periodontal disease is primarily the result of acidity of the mouth and the body.

Keep in mind that the word 'acidity' can have different meanings. We might speak of the flavour of a lemon as being acidic, yet in reality, lemon has an alkalising effect on the body by encouraging the pancreas to produce alkaline by-products that keep us healthy.

'So, you're saying I have unhealthy plaque *and* an unhealthy mouth?' Julian said.

'That's right. The harmful bacteria in your mouth have been flourishing, feeding on plaque and creating inflammation by making toxins that have irritated your gums and deteriorated your bone.'

'I don't understand,' Julian said. 'What would cause that acidity?'

'For you, dry mouth could certainly be a factor. This is a known side effect of a couple of the medications you're taking.

'Of course, if you're not taking good care of your teeth and gums, that would play a role too. Using toothpastes and mouthwashes made with harsh chemicals often does the most damage despite the best intentions. They destroy not only the harmful bacteria but also the beneficial bacteria – the whole population.

'But other factors can also contribute to acidity, like the food you eat, stress, smoking and drinking alcohol. If your immune system is compromised, it can predispose you to gum disease.

'You see, immunity, acidity and inflammatory diseases all have a two-way relationship with the oral microbiome – they can contribute to an imbalance in the mouth and can also be made worse by dental problems.'

From the Mouth to the Gut: A Single System

Did you know we swallow around two cups of saliva a day? This means that whatever is in our mouth – bacteria and the toxins they make, plus heavy metals and chemicals from dental materials like mercury (from amalgam fillings) and fluoride – will be swallowed and travel down into the stomach and the rest of the digestive system. There, they can disturb the balance of the gut microbiome, a distinct ecosystem of its own. Research has shown that bacteria in the mouth and in the stool overlap by forty-five percent.[41] Clearly, what goes on in our mouth, including gum disease, can affect the health of our gut.

> Did you know we swallow around two cups of saliva a day?

'To some extent, Julian, your stomach ulcer may be connected to the health of your gums.'

'You're kidding, right?' he said.

'Stomach ulcers are usually caused by a certain bacterium called *H. pylori*. Researchers have found these bacteria on the teeth and in the gum pockets of those who suffer from stomach ulcers.[42]

'So while people can receive treatment for the stomach ulcer and adjust their diet, if these bacteria persist in the mouth, they can be swallowed, reinfecting the stomach and causing more ulcers.'

It's not only stomach ulcers that have been found linked to harmful bacteria in the mouth, but also other inflammatory diseases of the gut, such as irritable bowel syndrome, Crohn's disease, ulcerative colitis and even colon cancers.[43] This discovery may one day allow us to detect a person's risk of diseases by looking in their mouth.

Research has also shown that harmful gut bacteria can affect the mouth, triggering bone loss around the teeth.[44] This highlights the two-way connection between the mouth and the gut. We know that in the case of acid reflux, the rise of acidic fumes from the stomach into the mouth can adversely affect oral health.[45]

Absorption through the Bloodstream: How Bacteria Invade the Body

In addition to the direct connection between the mouth and the gut, we also know that harmful oral bacteria and their toxins can be absorbed into the bloodstream through blood vessels in the mouth and from there, spread throughout the body.[46]

I brought up the topic with Julian.

'There's also a strong link between gum disease and cardiovascular disease.'[47]

'You're surprising me again,' Julian said.

For quite some time, we've known about the connection between oral bacteria and systemic illness. Dr Weston Price, a dentist from Canada, was one of the first medical practitioners to look into this link. You may have heard his name in regard to his research on the diets of certain native peoples in the 1920s. He found those cultures had exceptionally good dental health and overall health. You'll learn more about his research in the chapter on tooth decay.

Later in his career, Dr Price made another significant discovery while investigating root-canalled and dead teeth. He found a link between dental infections and heart problems. Later, he saw that this connection included other diseases like arthritis. In other words, he found evidence that bacteria in the mouth enter the bloodstream and affect other parts of the body.

Extensive research carried out over the past two decades consistently shows a strong link between cardiovascular disease and gum disease.[48] The risk of these conditions tends to rise in tandem.[49] People who suffer from periodontal disease are nearly twice as likely to develop heart disease.[50] The suspected link between these inflammatory diseases is the bacteria commonly found in both conditions. The harmful bacteria involved in gum disease make toxins that lead to inflammation of the gums (gingivitis) and degrade the natural barrier between the gums and the connective tissue within them. This breakdown of the barrier results in further inflammation.

Once the gums are inflamed, trouble begins.

'The bacteria and toxins in your mouth,' I told Julian, 'can be absorbed into the bloodstream very easily, especially if your gums are puffy and inflamed, as yours are. Everyday activities like chewing, brushing and flossing can push harmful bacteria into the gums and bloodstream, affecting various parts of the body, including the heart, brain and joints. These harmful invaders can take a world tour through your body, triggering inflammation wherever they settle.'

Have you heard of the term 'leaky gut', which proposes that undigested food particles, bacteria and toxins in the digestive tract can pass through the intestinal wall and enter the bloodstream? You can think of leaky gums in the same way, where harmful bacteria and toxins breach the gum tissue and enter the bloodstream.

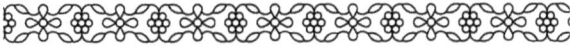

> These harmful invaders can take a world tour through your body, triggering inflammation wherever they settle.'

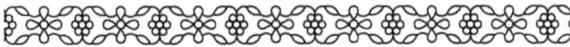

I explained to Julian that while in the bloodstream, the harmful bacteria that originated in the mouth can clump into tiny clots consisting of fats, immune cells and scar tissue. These clots are called atherosclerotic plaques, different from dental plaque.

'If a fragment of the clot breaks off,' I told Julian, 'and lodges in a blood vessel, it could obstruct the flow of blood to an important organ. If it makes its way to the brain, you could suffer a stroke. If it makes its way to the heart, it can cause a heart attack.'

Julian's eyes widened.

'So, what you're saying is that my unhealthy gums could have something to do with my stomach ulcer *and* my heart attack?'

'Yes, it's all connected. Julian, whatever blood flows around your teeth and gums flows around the rest of your body, through all of it.'

Protect Your Wellbeing by Nurturing Your Oral Health

We are now discovering that more and more diseases are connected to harmful bacteria in the mouth. A research paper titled the 'Gum–Gut Axis', published in 2021, unveiled a surprising finding: gum disease is linked to more than fifty diseases.[51]

Here are some of the places in the body where oral bacteria can potentially cause harm:

The Brain

Alzheimer's disease is linked to *P. Gingivalis*, a bacterium involved in gum disease. and Alzheimer's disease. When researchers examined brain samples of deceased patients who had Alzheimer's disease, this bacterium was discovered in their brain tissue. The bacteria are absorbed through the gums into the bloodstream, where they travel to the brain. Here, it is believed they cause Alzheimer's-like degeneration of the brain tissue.[52]

Dementia and periodontal disease are often seen hand in hand, especially among the elderly. The exact cause-and-effect relationship between the two is not yet fully understood. However, research suggests a strong association between periodontal health and cognitive function.[53]

Both Alzheimer's disease and dementia have been associated with brain atrophy, which in turn, has been linked to gum disease. Periodontitis and its resulting tooth loss can lead to a shrinkage of the hippocampus, the part of the brain critical for learning, emotional response and memory.[54] Hippocampal atrophy increases as periodontitis becomes more severe. Recent studies suggest that keeping teeth and gums healthy could help prevent brain shrinkage in adults of late middle age and older.

The Lungs

Due to the mouth's close proximity to the upper respiratory tract, bacteria that live in the mouth can easily be inhaled into the lungs. Especially at night, when our natural respiratory reflexes are reduced, it becomes more likely that we'll breathe in the contents of the mouth, including oral bacteria. These bacteria can then find their way into the lungs, which have their own distinct microbiome. This exchange of microbes between the mouth and the lungs can potentially impact respiratory health. Bacteria in the mouth have no place in the lungs and can cause harm, making us more susceptible to conditions such as chronic obstructive pulmonary disease (COPD), pneumonia and potentially, even lung cancer.[55]

The Joints

Rheumatoid arthritis is an autoimmune condition characterised by joint inflammation and pain. 'Autoimmune' means the body's immune system turns on itself. Studies have found the presence of harmful oral bacteria in the fluid surrounding the affected joints. While the exact role of oral bacteria in the development of arthritis is not yet fully understood, their presence suggests a potential link between oral health and the progression of this autoimmune disease.[56]

Metabolism and Hormones

Diabetes and periodontitis are closely linked. Inflammation in the mouth can give rise to systemic inflammation, which, in turn, can elevate blood glucose levels, increasing the risk of diabetes.[57] Conversely, diabetics are more vulnerable to infections, making them more likely to suffer from periodontitis.[58] The interaction between these two conditions is bidirectional, with each influencing the other and potentially exacerbating their effects.

Obesity is a growing global epidemic, and its association with an increased risk of various diseases is well established. An interesting connection exists between obesity and periodontitis.[59] The presence of gum disease leads to systemic inflammation, which can impact metabolism and hinder efforts to maintain a healthy body weight. Conversely, people who are overweight or obese have a higher likelihood of developing periodontitis.[60]

The Kidneys

When considering oral health, it's not often that we associate it with the health of our kidneys. Research shows, however, that periodontitis can cause inflammation of the kidneys and potentially kidney failure.[61]

Conception and Pregnancy

Periodontal disease can affect fertility and reproductive health. In women, the presence of periodontal disease can increase the difficulty of conception and elevate the risks of preterm birth, pre-eclampsia and low birth weight in babies.[62] It's important to note that the impact of periodontitis extends beyond women. Men with periodontal disease have been found to experience testicular dysfunction and a higher likelihood of male infertility.[63] These connections emphasise the significance of oral health in the broader context of reproductive wellbeing for both men and women.

What should we take away from all this? Taking care of our oral health really means we're taking care of our overall health.

'Okay, I get it,' Julian said. 'I have gum disease, it's serious and it could be affecting my health. So, what should I do?'

'First, we must deal with that loose tooth. Unfortunately, it will need to be extracted.'

'Oh, that's hard to accept,' he said, shifting in his chair. 'I thought you said the tooth was okay.'

'It is,' I said. 'The problem has to do with the

supporting structures around the tooth. Think of it this way: Your tooth is like a fencepost, and the gums and bone around it are like the soil holding the post in. If the soil level goes down, as yours has done, the post becomes loose.

'The good news is that moving forward, we can work on keeping you from losing more teeth.'

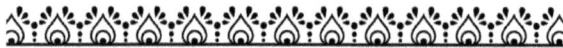

> What should we take away from all this? Taking care of our oral health means we're taking care of our overall health.

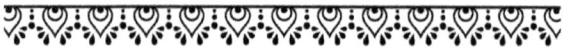

After I extracted Julian's tooth and cleaned out the bone socket around it, we scheduled a follow-up appointment for him to begin his journey to better oral health.

My hygienist carried out a detailed cleaning around Julian's teeth, known as deep scaling and root planing. She removed the plaque and calculus (tartar) on the surface of Julian's teeth and in the deep pockets of his gums that couldn't be reached by brushing and flossing.

With this deep cleaning, Julian's biofilm, or plaque build-up, was disrupted, exposing the area around his teeth and gums to oxygen, which destroyed the anaerobic bacteria living there. As the harmful bacteria were eliminated, Julian experienced a reduction in gum inflammation.

The root planing procedure resulted in a smoother root surface, which helped in the healing and reattachment of his gums to his teeth. This smoother surface also reduced the likelihood of plaque and calculus attaching to the teeth in the future.

I designed a customised oral care plan for Julian that emphasised the importance of cleaning his mouth not only before bed but also as soon as he wakes up in the morning, ideally within three minutes of rising. I guided him through the proper cleaning sequence, starting with brushing, followed by cleaning between the teeth, tongue cleaning and finally, rinsing with an oil-based herbal mouthwash.

Next, I looked at the oral care products Julian was using. I advised him to switch to a natural toothpaste without foaming agents or chemicals. The mouthwash he was swishing with contained a cocktail of artificial colourings, alcohol and fluoride. As a natural, alternative way to freshen his breath, I suggested he try some common herbs and spices.

Fighting Bad Breath, Naturally

Throughout history, cultures worldwide have explored and experimented with natural ways to achieve fresh breath.

In ancient Egypt, a common practice for freshening breath involved boiling aromatic ingredients such as cinnamon, myrrh and frankincense to create a mouthwash with refreshing properties.

The Romans ate parsley, which is still recognised as a breath freshener today. In the Middle East, cloves and sticks like miswak were chewed on, serving both as toothbrushes and breath fresheners.[64] In India, a common breath freshener and digestive aid to nibble on after a meal is 'Mukhwas', derived from the Sanskrit words *mukh* (mouth) and *vaas* (smell). This colourful blend is made of fragrant ingredients such as fennel, coconut, coriander seeds, sesame seeds and anise. It's often infused with essences of rose or mint. Perhaps you've seen a small dish of Mukhwas at Indian restaurants?

Most of the herbs and spices described below not only freshen breath and increase saliva production but also aid digestion, providing an added benefit not found in chemically based mouthwashes.

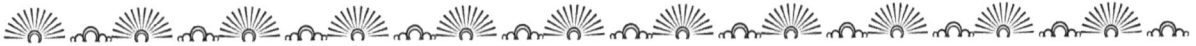

WHY DO I HAVE BAD BREATH?

- What's going on in your mouth? Poor oral hygiene, gum disease, tooth decay, infected tonsils, tonsil stones in the throat and tongue bacteria build-up can contribute to bad breath.
- What's going on in your body? Certain medical conditions, such as respiratory infections, gastrointestinal disorders and liver or kidney diseases can result in bad breath.
- What's going on in your lifestyle? Smoking, dry mouth and certain foods and beverages like garlic and coffee can cause unpleasant breath odour.

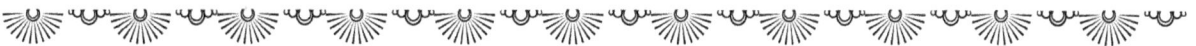

Nature's Breath Fresheners

Mint, in the form of peppermint or spearmint, is a universally associated flavour commonly found in toothpastes, mouthwashes and breath-freshening sweets known as 'mints'. Its use, however, spans through history and various cultures. In Morocco, mint tea is often served after a meal to freshen the breath and aid digestion. In my grandmother's garden, there was always a mint plant. She would not only add mint to her morning chai but would also pluck a few leaves to chew on after a meal. She understood the mouth-freshening properties of this herb and its support for digestion. Whether enjoyed as a tea or chewed directly, mint has always been a popular choice for breath freshening.

Green Cardamom was known as the 'Queen of Spices' in ancient India. It has a pleasant fragrance and taste. Even today, it is used in modern India to freshen breath and moisten the mouth. By placing a green cardamom pod, about the size of a pea, under your tongue and letting it mix with your saliva, you can experience its sweet taste and pleasing scent.

Fennel, a celery-like vegetable with a distinct liquorice flavour, offers breath-freshening properties. Chewing on fennel seeds not only freshens the breath but also stimulates saliva flow and reduces acidity in the mouth. The fibrous nature of fennel seeds also acts as a natural teeth cleanser.

According to both ancient Chinese Medicine and modern research, chewing fennel seeds has been found to reduce plaque formation and prevent gum disease.[65] You can chew on as little as a half teaspoon. I keep a jar of seeds at work so that if my mouth gets dry during the day (so common with wearing a mask) or I want to freshen my breath, I'll take a pinch of fennel seeds and chew on them.

Cinnamon and clove are great breath fresheners and are commonly used in natural toothpastes and mouthwashes for their refreshing properties. Placing a cinnamon stick or clove bud in your mouth allows it to soften with saliva and release its sweet and aromatic fragrance, helping to freshen your breath naturally.

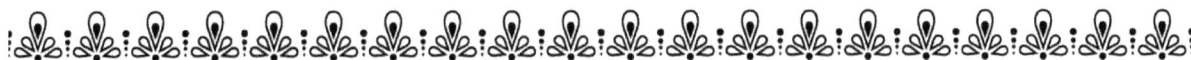

CREATE YOUR OWN AYURVEDIC MOUTHWASH

By combining just four natural ingredients, you can create a traditional Ayurvedic mouthwash that targets harmful oral bacteria.

Papaya and ginger reduce gum inflammation[66] and are beneficial for dry mouth.[67] Triphala, containing amla, which is rich in vitamin C, reduces plaque and gum inflammation.[68] Coconut oil, with its anti-bacterial properties, lubricates and moistens the mouth.[69]

This combination provides a powerful and natural solution for maintaining strong and healthy gums.

Ingredients

½ cup extra virgin organic coconut oil

1 tsp. triphala powder

5 drops ginger root essential oil

3 drops papaya seed oil

To prepare this Ayurvedic mouthwash, simply mix the ingredients together and store in a jar. When ready to use, take one teaspoon of the oil blend and place it in your mouth. If the oil solidifies in the jar, it will melt upon contact with the warmth of your mouth.

Later in the book, I will guide you on how to incorporate your mouthwash into your oral care routine.

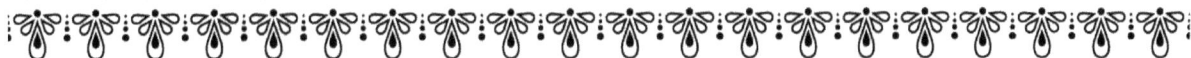

Just the Right Mouthwash

I explained to Julian that although his mouthwash might give temporary relief to his bad breath, in the long run, it could do more harm than good. Using an antiseptic-like mouthwash is comparable to taking an antibiotic every day to 'clean' the gut. It would ultimately strip the mouth not only of harmful bacteria but also of the beneficial ones that keep breath fresh and gum disease at bay. I recommended he either make his own mouthwash (see recipe above) or purchase one with more natural ingredients.

What Julian Is Doing Today

I proposed that Julian incorporate traditional Ayurvedic ingredients into his oral care routine. These natural ingredients, such as cinnamon, clove, cardamom, coconut oil, fennel, liquorice, mint, neem, tulsi and turmeric, have powerful healing properties and can effectively combat the harmful bacteria associated with gum disease; so too, with the Ayurvedic formula Triphala, which in Sanskrit means 'three fruits'. Triphala is a blend of bibhitaki, haritaki and amla (Indian gooseberry).

'You can also take these ingredients as teas,' I told him. 'It's like using a mouthwash throughout the day.'

Following Julian's deep cleanings, we set up regular dental check-ups to monitor the health of his gums and the bone around his teeth. My hygienist will continue to provide routine periodontal cleanings for Julian and offer guidance to ensure he remains comfortable with his new oral hygiene practices.

Equipped with the right oral care tools and specific botanicals suitable for his oral health needs, Julian now diligently follows his personal Dinacharya. He takes pride in the structured and precise order of his daily oral hygiene ritual, knowing that it contributes to the overall wellbeing of his mouth and body.

He has also extended the principles of Dinacharya to various aspects of his life. He has established a soothing night-time routine that helps reduce his stress. And he's adjusted his eating patterns with the natural rhythm of the day, focusing on eating plenty of fresh fruits, vegetables, healthy fats and proteins. As a result, his gut health has significantly improved, bringing him greater overall health.

As an adjunct to his improved diet, I recommended that Julian incorporate supplements specifically beneficial for gum and bone health.

6 Nutrients for Healthy Gums

1. Vitamin C is essential for healthy gums because of its role in forming collagen, which makes up the connective tissue in our gums, bones and teeth. Before the 19th century, sailors undertaking long sea voyages frequently faced a scarcity of fresh fruits and vegetables, resulting in a lack of adequate vitamin C intake. Since our bodies cannot store this water-soluble vitamin, it must be replenished on a daily basis. As a consequence of vitamin C deficiency, the

sailors developed scurvy, a condition characterised by muscle weakness, increased susceptibility to bruising, impaired wound healing and, notably, swollen and inflamed gums. The condition progressed to the point where their teeth would loosen and eventually fall out.

We now know so much about the health benefits of vitamin C, an essential for a healthy immune system. If you're low in this vitamin, you're more likely to develop gum disease.[70]

Topping the list of foods with the highest amount of vitamin C is amla. Revered in Ayurveda as an 'oral rebuilder', one tiny amla berry contains 20–30 times more vitamin C than an orange. Because amla is a sour fruit and often hard to find, many people prefer to take it in powder form or as part of the Ayurvedic herb, Triphala, which is also beneficial for gut health.

Fresh fruits and vegetables are good food sources of vitamin C including guava, bell peppers, oranges, strawberries and broccoli.

2. Coenzyme Q10 is a natural antioxidant produced by the body. It provides us with energy, promotes heart health, boosts the immune system and has been found to support healthy gums.[71] As we age, and if we have specific diseases, our body's natural CoQ10 production diminishes. I recommend taking CoQ10 in a chewable form, which allows for direct absorption into the gums while in the mouth, followed by swallowing for systemic benefit.[72] Food sources rich in CoQ10 include fatty fish, organ meats, soybeans, nuts, seeds and several vegetables, like broccoli. For patients who have gum disease, I strongly advise taking both vitamin C and CoQ10 as supplements.

3. Probiotics are often associated with improving gut health, but certain strains can also benefit oral health. Given that periodontal disease is linked to an imbalance of harmful bacteria, incorporating bacteria-rich fermented foods such as cultured yoghurt, sauerkraut or kimchi, or taking a probiotic supplement can help establish a healthy balance of beneficial bacteria in both the mouth[73] and the gut because the two ecosystems are interconnected.

As a child, when I had an upset stomach, my grandmother would prepare lassi, a traditional probiotic drink from India. It consists of cultured yoghurt mixed with water, cumin and salt – a simple Ayurvedic remedy (and a delicious drink) that remains popular today.

Researchers have discovered that probiotics can also reduce bad breath. They speculate it's because probiotics can prevent the breakdown of amino acids and proteins in the mouth and gut, which are responsible for the unpleasant odour we commonly associate with bad breath. [74]

4. Vitamin D is not only essential for the health of our immune system, muscles and bones, it also plays a significant role in oral health. Its antimicrobial properties, anti-inflammatory effects and ability to support bone health make it beneficial for our teeth and gums.[75] Vitamin D deficiency is widespread, so it's advisable to check your vitamin D levels through a blood test and, if necessary, increase sun exposure or take supplements.[76] Fish and eggs are good food sources of vitamin D.

5. Omega-3 fatty acids are beneficial for gum health, as they reduce inflammation, bleeding and swelling. Incorporating foods rich in Omega-3s, such as fatty fish, flaxseeds and walnuts into your diet, or taking a fish oil supplement, can support gum health.[77] Ayurveda's clarified butter, ghee, is also a rich source of Omega-3 fatty acids.

6. Zinc is an essential mineral that reduces inflammation and maintains healthy gums. Ensuring an adequate intake of zinc through sources such as nuts and seeds, legumes, dairy, eggs and whole grains can help support gum

health and reduce the risk of developing periodontal disease.[78]

I'm pleased to report that Julian has become more mindful of his oral health. He appreciates the flavours of the herbs and spices incorporated into his oral care products. With retirement providing him ample time, Julian has delved into researching the medicinal properties of herbs, spices and food. He is experimenting with various botanical ingredients in his diet as well as in his oral care products. Inspired by Julian, his wife has also embraced her own daily oral care routine.

Julian now has a deep appreciation for the significant impact that oral health can have on overall wellbeing. He recognises the importance of regular dental visits, which extend beyond mere cosmetic purposes. Julian now schedules those clinic visits months apart, not years, just as he does with his cardiologist, who has seen a marked improvement in his overall health.

Not only is Julian's mouth healthier, but his breath is fresher and his sense of taste has improved as a result of his new oral care practices. All of these changes have given Julian a great appreciation for the ancient wisdom of Ayurveda and how it can be applied to modern life.

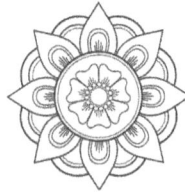

CHAPTER 4

TOOTH DECAY

There's More to Preventing Cavities than Brushing and Flossing

My next patient is Ruby, a healthy thirty-four-year-old mother of three young children – twin sons who are two and a daughter, four.

As well as her full-time role as a mother, Ruby has a part-time job as a yoga teacher. She's looking forward to increasing the number of classes she offers when her children are older.

Ruby is here for a routine check-up and hygiene appointment, which she diligently schedules and keeps every six months. My hygienist has carried out a professional cleaning and taken some X-rays after seeing a few suspicious areas on Ruby's teeth.

Now, it's my turn to check Ruby's mouth. And to break the news.

'I'm sorry, Ruby, but I can see from your X-rays that there's some decay between your teeth. I'll look more closely when I check your mouth, but it certainly appears you have a few cavities that will need fillings.'

'What! How could I have cavities? You know how well I look after my teeth. I brush and floss morning and night *and* use a fluoride toothpaste! And I don't eat many sweets at all. I thought it was people who ate sugar and didn't clean their teeth that got cavities.'

'I can see why you'd think that,' I said. 'Most

of us do. It goes back to one of the original theories of tooth decay.'

Back in 1890, a dentist by the name of Dr Willoughby D. Miller introduced the 'Acidogenic' hypothesis of tooth decay, a scientific opinion that has been around ever since.[79]

It's a fancy term for a process that's quite simple: Certain bacteria in dental plaque feed on sugars and refined carbohydrates in the mouth, then go on to make acids that 'demineralise' or 'melt' the enamel, the protective layer covering the tooth's outer surface.

Scientists have discovered the main bacterium involved in tooth decay: *Streptococcus mutans*.[80] We can try to keep this harmful bacterium under control by brushing, flossing and limiting sugar consumption, the standard recommendation dentists worldwide make and what I was taught at dental school.

The basis of Dr Miller's theory was the idea that a tooth is an inert mineral structure that, when exposed to bacteria and acids, deteriorates and erodes away over time. Initially, this starts out as a loss of some of the surface enamel, but as it progresses, a hole will eventually form in the tooth when the weakened enamel caves in. This hole is what we refer to as a cavity.

What we see, though, is that even people who don't eat a lot of sugar and do brush and floss every day, like Ruby, still develop cavities. This means Dr Miller's theory doesn't fully explain why dental decay is one of the most common non-communicable diseases on the planet. 'Non-communicable' means it isn't contagious. You can't pass it on by sharing a glass.[81]

'Sugar on your teeth,' I told Ruby, 'along with poor dental hygiene, can certainly contribute to decay. Over two billion people in the world have at least one cavity.[82] You're not alone, Ruby.'

'But how can I be one of those people when I do everything right?'

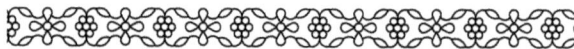

> What we see, though, is that even people who don't eat a lot of sugar and do brush and floss every day, like Ruby, still develop cavities.

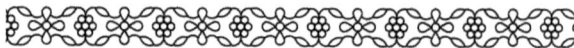

'Many factors can contribute to tooth decay. I'd like to get to the underlying causes of yours so we can prevent more from developing.'

'Yes, please. What do we do?'

'First, let me ask you a few questions. I know your children are young. Were they all breastfed?'

'Yes, they were. Not that nursing twins was easy.'

'I'm sure. And the children weren't born that far apart, right?'

'My daughter was about eighteen months old when I discovered I was pregnant with the twins,' Ruby said.

'It's possible the pregnancies and breastfeeding depleted your body of important minerals and nutrients. Have you heard of Dr Weston Price, the dentist who studied the diets of people who lived primitively?'

'I think so,' Ruby said. 'Isn't he the guy who said we should eat organ meats and soup made with animal bones? I couldn't do that. I'm a vegetarian.'

'That's a common misunderstanding. His point was that the healthiest people have a high level of nutrition, something we've lost today. Most of the principles of traditional diets can be adopted even if you're a vegetarian or vegan.'

A Look at Our Ancestors

In the 1920s, a few years after Dr Miller presented his research, Dr Weston Price, a Canadian dentist working in the United States, became interested in finding out more about what caused tooth decay. He suspected that changes in the American diet and lifestyle could have something to do with the rise in cavities he was seeing.

Dr Price had come to learn of certain primitive cultures around the world who were living away from modern civilisation and subsisting on their native, ancestral diet. What interested him was that these people had exceptional dental and general health. Intrigued, he set off travelling to those places to find out more. He visited the First Nations people of Australia, Pacific Islanders, South American Indians and many others.

He saw that these people were very healthy – not only physically but also mentally and spiritually. They didn't suffer the same level of dental decay and chronic diseases seen in more modern parts of the world.

When he examined their teeth, he found them strong, healthy and sitting perfectly spaced in their wide jaws. Think about it for a moment: These people lived primitively. There were no electric toothbrushes or dentists in sight. When these same people were introduced to a modern diet over time, their jaws and airways narrowed, and they developed gum disease and dental decay.[83]

'What Dr Price found,' I told Ruby, 'was that these people all ate nutrient-dense and natural, organic whole foods. Their grains were freshly ground, and the plants they ate were rich in minerals. No vegetable oils, white sugar, white flour or processed foods.

'They included nuts, sprouted seeds, milk, eggs, cheeses, meats and seafood for protein. Sweets, even natural ones, were rarely consumed and only on special occasions.'

'We eat a very healthy diet at home. No junk food. It's only when the children go to birthday parties that we allow them a treat,' Ruby said.

'I'm sure that's true and that you're doing your best, but modern farming practices have stripped our soils of many nutrients and loaded our food with chemicals. A tomato today is very different nutritionally than one our grandmothers would have eaten.'

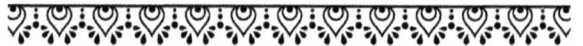

The people Dr Price studied had a deep reverence for the land and dedicated considerable time and energy to maintain and enhance the quality of their growing soil. They also had the wisdom to know how plant medicines could heal. Some tribes in Africa, for example, knew how to prevent goitre by eating iodine-rich food such as seaweed.

Due to the depletion of nutrients in modern soils, it has become challenging for us to get the full spectrum of essential vitamins and minerals we need, especially the fat-soluble ones. For strong teeth that are resistant to decay, we need vitamins A, D and K2. These vitamins work synergistically with each other.

Vitamin A helps in the absorption of vitamin D,[84] which, in turn, helps us absorb calcium.[85] Vitamin K2 is one of three types of vitamin K. It helps vitamin D move calcium and other minerals into the teeth and bones.[86] Dr Price referred to vitamin K2 as 'Activator X', which he found was abundant in the diets of the healthy people he studied. They consumed high-vitamin butter, cod liver oil, seafood and animal organs rich in fat.

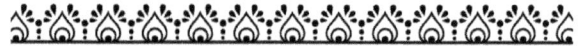

> A tomato today is very different nutritionally than one our grandmothers would have eaten.

Emerging research also suggests that vitamin E may help prevent enamel erosion, protecting against tooth decay.[87]

If we look to Ayurveda, we find that ghee, a nutritious clarified butter, is rich in all these very vitamins.

Ghee: Ancient Elixir for Good Health

As mentioned in the Ayurveda chapter, ghee has been revered as a sacred food by generations of people in India since ancient times. It continues to have a prominent place in Indian kitchens to this day.

Ghee is made by simmering unsalted butter over low heat until the milk solids separate from the oil.

In addition to its dental benefits, ghee is also good for bone health. Interestingly, in Ayurvedic medicine, teeth are considered part of bone tissue, so it makes sense that whatever nutrients support our bones will be good for our teeth.

Ghee also supports gut health because it contains butyric acid, an anti-inflammatory that promotes the growth of good bacteria.[88] From an Ayurvedic perspective, ghee supports Agni, our digestive fire.

With its high content of monounsaturated Omega-3s, the good fats, ghee can also reduce high cholesterol levels and support heart health.[89] It can even help with weight loss.[90]

This Ayurvedic butter can be eaten directly or used for cooking, even at high temperatures. And because the lactose and casein have solidified and been discarded, you can eat ghee if you're lactose intolerant. Despite its many health benefits, ghee should be taken in moderation. It's recommended not to take more than one to two teaspoons a day.

Why not make your own ghee using my grandmother's recipe below? To this day, I can recall the delicious, sweet aroma that filled her home when she made ghee. That same scent permeates my kitchen when I make my own ghee, transporting me back in time to treasured moments with her.

Dr Price also found that people living on traditional diets made sure to eat some form of fermented foods rich in beneficial bacteria, either vegetables like kimchi, sauerkraut and pickles, or dairy products like cultured yoghurt, lassi and kefir. Ancient wisdom must have had an innate knowledge of the importance of fermented foods and understood that the probiotics they contain are necessary for good gut health.

HOW TO MAKE GOLDEN GHEE

1. Heat

Place 1 kg of unsalted butter (if possible, organic and from grass-fed cows) into a medium-sized pot with a heavy bottom. Place the pot over low to medium heat depending on the temperature settings of your stove so that the ghee doesn't burn.

2. Simmer

Once the butter has melted, reduce the heat to a low setting and let the butter simmer for 15–20 minutes. Now would be the perfect time to pause for a moment, take a few deep breaths and savour the ghee's rich, sweet smell and its deep, golden colour.

You'll notice white curds on the surface of the butter as it continues to simmer, and you'll hear the liquid make a popping sound. After the curds have turned a tan colour and the popping has slowed down, turn off the heat and let the ghee cool for 30 minutes, until it's just warm.

3. Strain

Use a cheesecloth to strain the ghee into a clean glass jar. Discard the curds collected in the cloth and at the bottom of the pan.

Store the ghee at room temperature and enjoy.

Eating Well and Living Well

In each culture Dr Price studied, he observed that the native diet was in alignment with the seasons. It included periods of under-eating and fasting, either as rituals or due to natural shortages of food. These days, we call this intermittent fasting.

Fresh air, sunlight and daily physical exercise were also common to their lives.

What these people ate, how they ate and how they lived tapped into primitive wisdom that supported their health and happiness.

To clarify, Dr Price did not believe all traditional rituals were inherently good and that modern civilisation was entirely bad.

However, he did emphasise the importance of understanding and preserving traditional wisdom while also recognising the benefits of advancements in modern society.

The philosophies of Ayurveda place importance on eating nutrient-rich foods and living with an understanding of the rhythms of nature, practices very much in line with Dr Price's findings.

'In many of the cultures Dr Price studied,' I told Ruby, 'they carefully spaced the births of their children and had special diets, sometimes even for the father, to support conception, pregnancy and lactation. They knew what nutrients they needed and how to get them. In our modern world, it can be hard to manage all that.'

'But I eat so healthy,' Ruby said.

'I have no doubt you eat well,' I said. 'It's possible, Ruby, that these cavities could have developed because of a deficiency of essential vitamins and minerals during pregnancy and breastfeeding, when a large amount of nutrients are directed towards the baby's growth and development.

'A simple blood test could check your vitamin and mineral levels, especially vitamins D and C, calcium, potassium and phosphorus. Do you have a doctor who could look into this?'

Ruby smiled. 'I've just started seeing an integrative doctor who has a holistic approach. I found out about her from another yoga teacher.'

'Great,' I said. 'Now that we've addressed the nutritional aspects of decay, let's look into other causes that might be contributing to your cavities.'

Tooth Decay Is a Systemic Disease, Not Just One of the Mouth

A few decades after the work of Dr Price, Dr Ralph Steinman, a dentist at Loma Linda University in California took a fresh look and delved deeper into the Acidogenic theory of tooth decay.[91]

He noticed that some people, even those with poor oral hygiene, just don't get cavities. I've observed this throughout my career as well.

Dr Steinman wondered what other factors might contribute to, or even cause, cavities. He also suspected that teeth had a way of protecting themselves from decay.

Over the course of forty years, he conducted numerous experiments. He injected sugar and processed foods directly into the stomachs of one-half of a group of rats and healthy, nutritious food into the stomachs of the other half. Even though none of the rats had food placed directly into their mouths, the group that was injected with sugar and processed foods developed tooth decay, and the group that received more nutritious food did not. In essence, the process of decay started in the stomach, not in the mouth.

Dr Steinman also experimented with adding calcium and phosphorous, the main minerals that make up a tooth's structure, to the diet of the rats fed sugar and processed food. Amazingly, their decay rate decreased by eighty per cent, which tells us we need minerals for strong teeth.

Still not satisfied, Dr Steinman called upon an endocrinologist he knew, a medical doctor specialising in the body's glands and the hormones they make. Together, they removed the parotid glands (the major salivary glands located near the jaw) in the group of rats receiving the healthy food. These rats developed decay, telling us that our endocrine system (our hormones) plays a vital role in preventing tooth decay. Stress can disrupt our hormonal balance, which in turn, can increase our susceptibility to cavities.

Even more interesting, Dr Steinman found that teeth are not static, inert mineral structures. They're a sophisticated, living system.

Just like other organs in our body, they receive nourishment and expel waste through their own blood, nerve and lymphatic supply, which we call the 'dentinal fluid transport system.' If this fluid is healthy and flowing well, the tooth is well nourished from the inside out and protected from tooth decay.

Both Dr Price's findings and Dr Steinman's research show us that the health of our teeth involves more than avoiding sugar and brushing our teeth.

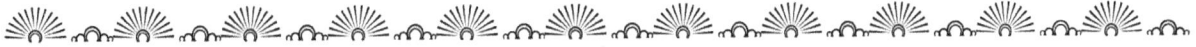

WHY DO I HAVE CAVITIES?

Although we're still learning about decay and will certainly know even more in future years, today we understand that decay can be caused by multiple factors. These include:

- poor oral hygiene
- excess sugar consumption
- nutritional deficiencies
- dry mouth
- stress
- poor digestive health
- poor immunity
- hormonal imbalances.

If any of these areas are weak, from poor diet to gut issues to stress, the flow of dentinal fluid to and from the teeth is disrupted and the outer layer of the tooth becomes vulnerable to harmful bacteria, toxins and acids. This sets the scene for decay to start.

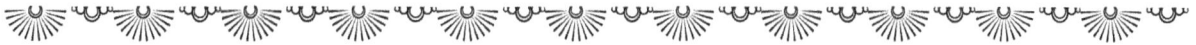

I had more questions for Ruby.

'With all you have going on, you must be very busy. Do you get enough sleep?'

'No, not really, but coffee does help me get through the day.'

'How many cups do you usually have?' I asked.

'Maybe three or four.'

'And does your mouth get dry?'

'Sometimes," she said, 'but chewing gum helps. I buy one with xylitol from the health food store because I read it's good for your teeth.'

'I'm sure the coffee helps you keep your energy levels up during the day, but the caffeine could be affecting your absorption of calcium. Alcohol and soft drinks do the same thing.'

'I don't go for fizzy drinks and have hardly any alcohol. Giving up my coffee is out of the question.'

'Perhaps you could gradually reduce your coffee intake and swap it for some herbal tea? There are so many that not only taste delicious but can also reduce the acidity in your mouth and keep it hydrated. To protect against the main bacteria involved in tooth decay, *S mutans*, I recommend tulsi,[92] liquorice,[93] clove,[94] fennel[95] and cardamom.[96]

'And to help remineralise your teeth, you could include herbs like moringa[97] or ginger.'[98]

I explained to Ruby that coffee would not only affect her calcium absorption but would also act as a diuretic, pulling water out of her mouth and making it feel dry.

'What does a dry mouth have to do with cavities?' Ruby asked.

'When our mouth is dry, it means we don't have enough saliva. Our saliva washes our mouth all day long, removing harmful bacteria and nourishing our gums and teeth. A dry mouth is the perfect environment for decay to develop.

'And I know that chewing gum can feel like it helps keep your mouth moist,' I told her, 'but I don't recommend it, even if it contains xylitol. There's no question that xylitol can reduce the amount of acid-producing bacteria in the mouth.[99] It's the act of chewing gum that concerns me.'

'Why?' she asked.

'When we chew, our brain thinks food will be passing down from our mouth to our stomach soon, so it sends a signal to the stomach to make hydrochloric acid.

'We need hydrochloric acid to break down proteins in the stomach, but if we're constantly chewing without swallowing, acidity can build up in the stomach and lead to issues like acid reflux and stomach ulcers.'

Reflux, in particular, is damaging to the mouth because it makes it more acidic, opening the door to issues like teeth erosion, cavities, bad breath and gum disease.

Chewing gum can also cause bloating because as we chew, we're taking in small amounts of air.

From an Ayurvedic perspective, the imbalance created by excess hydrochloric acid or air in the stomach weakens Agni.

And if you're a teeth grinder, chewing gum can put an extra demand on your jaw muscles, making them feel even more sore. The constant compression can cause tension headaches and lead to problems with the temporomandibular joints (TMJs).

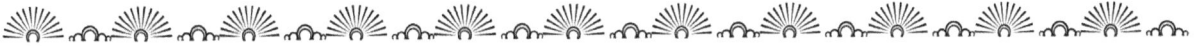

THE LIFE OF A CAVITY

During a cavity's early stages, it's possible you won't feel any sensitivity or pain, as was the case for Ruby. Nevertheless, decay has set in and can often be found by a dental hygienist or dentist. Sometimes we're able to see it as a brown or black spot that's soft or sticky when we probe it. Other times, it may not be visible to the naked eye. This is where X-rays can be helpful, especially for finding cavities between the teeth.

Once the decay has reached the dentine layer under the enamel, it will continue to spread and, in some cases, quite quickly, like rust through a car. This is because dentine is a softer and less resistant mineral than enamel.

If left untreated, the bacteria will continue to erode the mineral, eventually creating a cavity in the tooth. This cavity provides an opening for more bacteria and acids to penetrate deeper, approaching the pulp chamber, where the nerve of the tooth lives. This progression can lead to sensitivity and pain.

As the decay advances, it will eventually reach the nerve of the tooth, creating an infection that consumes the tooth's nutrients. Without these nutrients, the tooth loses its vitality and dies. At this stage, you may experience a toothache, but it's also possible to feel nothing at all.

When a tooth dies, the only available treatment options are an endodontic procedure, known as root canal treatment, or extraction of the tooth, neither of which is desirable.

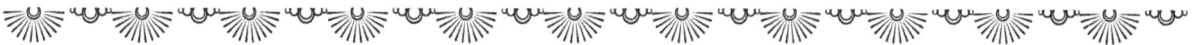

Can I Heal My Cavities Naturally?

'Okay, so I'll cut down on coffee and stop chewing gum if it will help,' Ruby said, 'but isn't there some way I can heal these cavities without having to get fillings? I've seen some toothpastes and vitamins on the internet saying that you can naturally repair a tooth without visiting the dentist.'

'Yes, in some cases, if the decay is in its very early stages,' I told her, 'and still in the outer layer of the tooth, the enamel. That's what dentists call 'early demineralisation'. It's essentially a pre-cavity, and in this situation, it might be possible to naturally remineralise the tooth surface.

'But in your case, Ruby, the decay has gone further. It's already spread into the dentine, which is harder to repair.'

The question Ruby posed is one I am often asked. While there are many bold claims on the internet about certain vitamins and supplements being able to naturally heal cavities, most of these claims are not supported by scientific evidence. If you have doubts or questions about the information you come across, please seek out research or scientific studies that can support the claims being made. Throughout my career, I've seen people who've placed their trust in such claims only to find themselves visiting my clinic for the first time with a severe toothache. Unfortunately, more often than not, they ended up needing treatment that was invasive and costly, and in some cases, resulted in the loss of the tooth.

I understand the reasoning behind this question: If it's possible to heal bones, then surely it's possible to heal teeth. After all, bones and teeth are made of the same minerals.

The difference lies in the fact that bones are within the body, where the internal environment maintains a relatively stable acid–alkaline balance. This environment favours the process of remineralisation and healing.

Teeth, on the other hand, are in the mouth, which can fluctuate in acidity. Every time we eat, the environment inside our mouth becomes acidic. An acidic environment is not conducive to tooth remineralisation.

While natural remedies are helpful in preventing and treating tooth decay in its very early stages, they should not replace professional dental treatment.

Natural Toothache Relief

A toothache can be extremely painful and even debilitating. Under such circumstances, resorting to pain medication may become an unavoidable necessity. Here is when we may truly appreciate the benefits of modern medicine.

Our ancestors, who did not have the anaesthetics and painkillers available to us today, possessed the knowledge that certain spices could help alleviate pain.

Here are some spices that have been used in ancient India for thousands of years and are known for their ability to relieve pain in the mouth:

Clove is a strong painkiller with a powerful numbing effect, making it a perfect remedy for toothaches. Its active ingredient is oil of eugenol, which gives us the classic smell of clove we know. Perhaps you've noticed this scent while visiting the dentist. Why? Because the benefits of clove oil are recognised even in modern dentistry, where it is used in many dental cements.

Not only does clove provide pain relief, it also supports dental health with its rich supply of calcium and high antioxidant levels. It's naturally antiseptic, antibacterial and antifungal, making it a great remedy for oral thrush (Candida).

I have childhood memories of my grandmother reaching for clove when she had a toothache. She would chew on a clove bud, crushing it to release the pain-relieving oil.

Cinnamon is another spice that can help alleviate dental pain. It can be used in the same way as clove.

Turmeric, a golden-coloured spice used in cooking all over Asia, can also relieve pain. Its active ingredient, curcumin, has long been recognised in Ayurveda for its powerful anti-inflammatory properties and its ability to heal wounds. These qualities make it perfect for soothing mouth ulcers, toothaches and post-extraction discomfort.

You can make a simple remedy by mixing one teaspoon of salt and one teaspoon of turmeric in half a cup of warm water, then swishing it in your mouth.

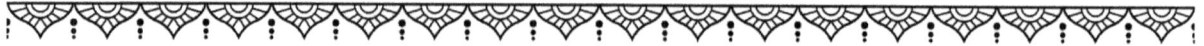

TOOTHACHE BLEND

Combine the ingredients below into a paste:

2 tbsp. ghee or coconut oil (warming the oil slightly can make it easier to blend the ingredients)
3 drops clove essential oil or 1 tsp. ground clove powder
3 drops turmeric essential oil or 1 tsp. turmeric powder

Soak a cotton ball in the mixture and place the cotton next to the sore tooth.

Repeat every four hours until you can be seen by your dentist.

Note: Please do not apply clove oil straight onto your gums. It is a potent oil and can cause irritation or ulceration if it comes into direct contact with gum tissue.

Although this remedy can provide temporary relief from dental pain, it is not intended to replace professional dental care. It is always advisable to consult a dentist for proper diagnosis and treatment.

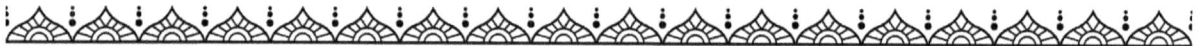

'Now, let's talk about your sleep deprivation, Ruby, and your stress levels. Stress makes a dry mouth worse and affects so much more. And good sleep is essential. Do you have a night-time ritual?

'For me,' I said, 'it's a twenty-minute soak in a warm bath or a warm oil massage followed by a shower. I switch off the phone, light a candle, play some calming music and relax.'

'With three kids? I hardly have any time for myself.'

Over the years, I've seen many women in situations similar to Ruby's.

They often find themselves overwhelmed,

juggling multiple responsibilities such as a career, childcare, managing finances and nurturing their relationships. They put everyone else's needs before their own, leaving little time and energy for self-care. On the outside, these women may appear strong and capable, but beneath the surface, they may be struggling.

'Ruby, I understand how busy you are. Can you find even an hour a week for yourself?'

Her eyes filled with tears, and she quickly looked down.

I reached out to touch her arm.

'You know, Ruby, Dr Price found that the health of the people he studied was not just about their diet but also their way of life. They were deeply connected to the natural world, followed the rhythms of day and night and prioritised restful sleep. They lived without the modern-day stresses we often face. It's important for us to find ways to bring some of these elements into our lives, even if it's in small doses, for our own balance and wellness.

'I can help you design a plan to care for your teeth to prevent more cavities. And as part of that plan, I'm asking you to think of some small ways you can slow down and create space for your own self-care. Spend some time in nature, whether it's in the garden, at the beach or in a park. Take time

for yourself, away from the daily stresses and demands of your busy life.'

Ruby didn't reply, but I could tell we had turned a corner.

Oral Care for the Decay-Prone

For Ruby's oral care, I suggested she select products free from harsh chemicals and instead focus on natural ingredients, including a fluoride-free toothpaste infused with the herbs and spices we discussed earlier for her teas. As an alternative to fluoride, I also recommended she choose a toothpaste containing hydroxyapatite, an ingredient known for its ability to remineralise enamel and strengthen teeth.

Hydroxyapatite is a naturally occurring form of calcium and phosphate, which are the building blocks of our bones and teeth. It is referred to as 'biomimetic' because its composition closely resembles the natural hydroxyapatite found in our teeth and bones. As a result, our body recognises it and knows how to interact with it. When applied to the teeth, hydroxyapatite can support the remineralisation process by replenishing lost minerals and strengthening the tooth enamel. This biomimetic property is not only valuable for oral care but also extends to other areas of medicine like orthopaedics, where hydroxyapatite is used for bone healing and regeneration.

Better yet, it doesn't destroy the helpful bacteria in the mouth or disrupt the balance of the oral microbiome.

'And it's non-toxic and safe for children,' I told Ruby. 'Hydroxyapatite has been scientifically proven to remineralise tooth enamel.[100] It is more effective than fluoride in preventing cavities.'[101]

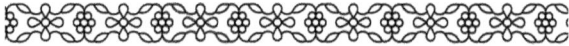

> When applied to the teeth, hydroxyapatite can support the remineralisation process by replenishing lost minerals and strengthening the tooth enamel.

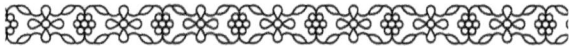

'I thought we needed fluoride in our toothpaste,' Ruby said. 'Although now that I think about it, I guess it didn't keep me from getting cavities.'

'Well, as we talked about, there are so many other factors involved in tooth decay,' I said.

'My concern with fluoride is that scientific research has begun to show that it's actually a toxin, especially at high levels.[102] It's not a vitamin or a nutrient. Our bodies don't need it to function. You will never be told that your health is compromised because you are deficient in fluoride.'

'You mean, fluoride's actually harmful?' Ruby said.

'It can be, in many ways. It depresses the thyroid gland by displacing iodine.[103] It can also calcify the pineal gland, that small gland in our brain responsible for producing melatonin, which regulates our sleep patterns.[104] The pineal is also known as the seat of the soul and is associated in Eastern spirituality with the concept of the third eye.'

'I know about the pineal gland from my yoga studies,' Ruby said. 'I had no idea it could be affected by fluoride.'

'Fluoride even reduces our intelligence,'[105] I said. 'And if your children swallow it, their teeth could eventually change from a smooth, natural look to a mottled white or brown. In some cases, the teeth can become pitted. This is called dental fluorosis. Instead of strengthening the teeth, fluoride can potentially weaken them.'[106]

'Okay, no more fluoride toothpaste for my family,' Ruby said. 'I'll buy one with hydroxyapatite instead.'

Is Fluoride the Magic Bullet?

When I qualified as a dentist in 1995, my first job as a new graduate was in the paediatric dentistry department of King's College School of Medicine and Dentistry in London, the university where I received my degree.

We saw children coming in with decayed teeth that needed fillings. As a preventative measure, we painted strong fluoride varnishes onto their teeth or placed trays in their mouths filled with a highly concentrated fluoride gel. Our aim was to strengthen their teeth and protect against future decay. When we saw these same children a few months later, they had new decay and more cavities. *Something wasn't working as expected,* I thought to myself.

What I did notice was the type of food these children were eating. At that time, King's College was in a low socio-economic area of South East London where perhaps the best dietary practices weren't observed. The children coming into the clinic were consuming bottles of sweetened fruit juices like Ribena, and also white-bread sandwiches and potato chips, or 'crisps' as we call them in the UK – all processed junk food with very little nutritional value.

This led me to think. *The reason these children are developing tooth decay lies deeper than having too many sweets. And if fluoride is so important for preventing tooth decay, then it certainly isn't working here. There must be more to this.*

And now we know there is. The studies of Neanderthal skulls and the findings of Dr Price confirm that teeth do not need fluoride to be strong and healthy. So many other factors are involved in the prevention of tooth decay.

When we look at countries such as Austria, Belgium, Finland, France, Germany and several others in Europe, we see they've stopped water fluoridation as a public health measure and yet have not witnessed an increase in their decay rate.

While fluoride is recommended by most dentists, I encourage you to carry out your own research and make an informed choice as to whether you choose to use fluoride.

'Now you've got me worried,' Ruby said. 'We've been using a fluoride toothpaste all these years.'

'Ayurveda has a way to detoxify fluoride from our bodies,' I told her, 'whether it's from toothpaste or drinking water. You can add turmeric, tulsi and aloe vera juice to your diet. They've all been scientifically proven to help remove fluoride from the body.'[107]

'Now, back to what we *do* want in your toothpaste. Another beneficial ingredient is clay.'

'Clay?' Ruby said. 'I've used it as a face mask before, but I didn't know it was good for the mouth too.'

'Clays are naturally antibacterial[108] and they can reduce acidity in the mouth, which is exactly what we want for a healthy oral microbiome.'

Throughout history, ancient civilisations like the Egyptians, African tribesmen, the First Nations people of Australia and North American Indians have used clays for both internal and external cleansing purposes. Known as the mud that heals, clays were prized by the Egyptians for their anti-inflammatory and antiseptic properties.

Drawing on this ancient knowledge, we can enrich our own dental care practices.

Bentonite clay[109] and kaolin are two types of clays found to have benefits for dental health. Bentonite clay is made from volcanic ash that has been weathered by the ocean over a long time. Kaolin is a white clay commonly known as China clay.

'I don't think I've ever really looked at a toothpaste ingredient list,' Ruby said. 'But I'll do that from now on.'

We arranged appointments for Ruby to have her cavities filled, and I helped her design her daily oral care routine. That included toothbrushing, followed by flossing, which was particularly important as Ruby had cavities between her teeth. I suggested that she apply a small amount of toothpaste to the biting surfaces of her teeth before flossing. That way, the floss would carry the hydroxyapatite down between her teeth, maximising its effectiveness.

After flossing, I advised her to clean her tongue and then finish by swishing with an oil-based mouthwash. This would help remove harmful bacteria and lubricate her mouth. I suggested looking for a mouthwash containing papaya or ginger, as they both help stimulate saliva production.

Ruby embraced my suggestions and was amazed that she can care for her oral health naturally. She's switched to a fluoride-free toothpaste containing natural, non-toxic ingredients like clove, cinnamon, liquorice, hydroxyapatite and bentonite clay.

'I love the taste,' she said, smiling. 'My daughter enjoys it too, and it gives me peace of mind to know it's not causing us any harm.'

She's also embarked on a journey of exploring herbal teas for oral health and has become quite the connoisseur. Researching and experimenting with different herbs like tulsi, moringa, liquorice and others, Ruby now has an impressive collection of teas. She takes pleasure in creating her own unique blends and enjoys the added benefits they bring to her oral wellbeing.

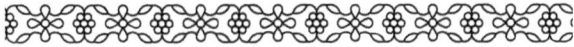

> She's switched to a fluoride-free toothpaste containing natural, non-toxic ingredients like clove, cinnamon, liquorice, hydroxyapatite and bentonite clay.

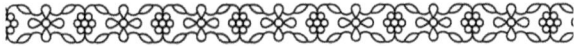

Despite her love of coffee, Ruby has made a conscious effort to limit her consumption during the day. Instead, she now enjoys her morning cup in solitude before her children wake up, appreciating the small moments of joy in her life. By swapping her coffee for herbal teas, she's noticed her mouth doesn't feel as dry, and she no longer needs to rely on chewing gum for relief.

With a few diet changes and supplements, Ruby also addressed some nutritional imbalances picked up in a routine blood test. She now includes calcium-rich sesame seeds and ghee in her diet to support her oral health.

Ruby started to explore Ayurveda as its true sister companion to her yoga practice and is amazed at the many ways Ayurveda can nurture her wellbeing. By incorporating simple Ayurvedic principles into her life, she has improved her health and the health of her family.

When I saw Ruby at her next check-up, I found her mouth was much healthier and there were no cavities.

I'm delighted our work together has enhanced Ruby's entire life, not just her oral health. And it all started with a few cavities.

Keep up the great work, Ruby!

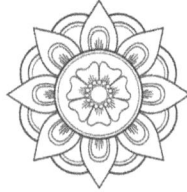

CHAPTER 5

STRESSED-OUT MOUTH

Clenching and Grinding: The Burden Our Teeth Bear

When my next patient of the day walked in, I immediately suspected she was a teeth grinder or, at the very least, a clencher. How could I tell? The jaw muscles in her cheeks, her masseters, were the giveaway.

They were bulging as if she'd been exercising them at the gym. Veena had come to see me because she could feel an uneven, rough area on one of her teeth.

'I'm worried the tooth might be chipped,' she said.

'Okay, we'll have a good look. Is anything else bothering you? I noticed you were rubbing the back of your neck.'

'My neck and back get so sore. I'm a hairdresser, so I guess it comes with the job. My shoulders have been tight too. And, I've been having a lot of headaches. I've been under so much stress.'

I was getting more information from Veena … and I hadn't even looked in her mouth!

'Tell me more about that stress,' I said. 'You'd be surprised at what stress can do to the body, even the mouth. It seems as though almost everyone is under some amount of stress these days.'[110]

'I'm sure they are,' she said, her jaw clenched tightly shut. Then tears began to slide down her cheeks.

'My husband passed away last year. I didn't

expect to become a widow so young. I'm only fifty-three.'

As the tears continued to flow, I passed Veena a box of tissues and put my hand on her shoulder.

'I'm so sorry,' I said.

After a minute she collected herself. 'I'm the one who's sorry. I seem to cry over anything these days.'

'Well, that's not just anything,' I said. 'Are you by any chance going through menopause?'

She inhaled deeply. 'Yes. For the past two years. So many hot flushes. I can't remember when I last slept well.'

'I see from your medical history form that you're taking an antidepressant. And you were recently diagnosed with leaky gut syndrome?'

Veena looked down and dabbed her eyes with a tissue. 'Yes, it's all too much,' she said.

'Well,' I said, 'let's take one thing off your mind – that tooth. I'm going to lie you back now and take a look.'

The Telltale Signs of Clenching and Grinding

The tooth in question was indeed chipped. It didn't have a filling, and I couldn't see any decay. Why had this tooth broken?

As I looked around the rest of Veena's mouth,

I could see the tips of her canines (also known as the 'eye' teeth) were worn down and looked flat instead of pointy. The chewing surfaces of her back teeth, the molars, also appeared flat. They were yellow, a sign that the enamel was wearing away, exposing the darker-coloured dentine underneath.

'Have you noticed any sensitivity to hot or cold foods or drinks?' I asked.

'Now that you mention it, yes! Especially when I drink my morning smoothie. I'm trying to lose some weight.'

I could see a few areas where Veena's gums had started to recede from her teeth. They also looked puffy, more like a necklace dangling from the teeth rather than a picture of the firm snugness of healthy gums.

Let me explain. Imagine a trip to the beach. You find a spot on the sand where you decide to settle and put up your umbrella. You push the pole deep into the sand and pat the sand firmly around it. Imagine the wind picks up and shakes the umbrella. The sand will be disrupted, will 'puff up' and move away from the pole. Now think of your tooth as that umbrella pole and your gum as the sand.

It's a common belief that gum recession is caused by brushing the teeth too hard. While this is true in many cases, another cause, often over-looked, is clenching and grinding. If I see only a couple of teeth where the gums have pulled away, it's telling me something else is going on. After all, it's unlikely that we're brushing just two teeth hard and not the others. More likely is that those two teeth are under heavy pressure, receiving that umbrella-shaking force I just described.

Our masseters are the main muscles we use when we chew, and they're one of the strongest muscles in the body when measured in terms of their strength per pound. Together with our other jaw muscles, our masseters are capable of exerting a pressure of up to twenty-five kilograms (fifty-five pounds) on our front teeth and up to ninety-one kilograms (two hundred pounds) on our back teeth![111]

This tremendous force not only causes the gums to recede, but it also wears down the tooth's enamel and can compress the tooth's nerve bundle at the base of the tooth. Imagine the nerve as an electrical power cord being repeatedly pressed under a heavy weight. Just as the power cord's insulation can be damaged or develop internal shorts, so the nerve becomes agitated, creating sensitivity in the tooth, particularly to cold.

Add to this tooth-pounding ability, the jaw's constant activity. The jaw is one of the only places in the body that doesn't fully rest while we're asleep.

Have you ever noticed that babies suckle in their sleep? It's a self-soothing action. Our jaws are active even when we're not. Now we begin to see the potential for trauma.

I say to my patients who clench or grind their teeth at night, 'It's like your jaw muscles are lifting weights every night when they should be resting!'

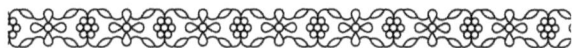

Clues inside and outside of Veena's mouth were leading me to believe she was grinding her teeth. Bulging masseter muscles, a sore neck, a chipped tooth, worn-down teeth, cold sensitivity and receding, puffed-up gums – all classic signs and symptoms of teeth grinding.

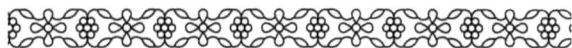

> I say to my patients who clench or grind their teeth at night, 'It's like your jaw muscles are lifting weights every night when they should be resting!'

Check for signs of clenching and grinding in your own mouth by simply looking in the mirror.

Squeeze your teeth tightly together and touch the muscles in front of your ears. These are your masseter muscles. Are they bulging? Do they feel hard? Tender? Sore?

Next, look inside your mouth:

- Shine a light on your teeth and look for any crack lines running from the gum to the biting edge. If your teeth are under a lot of force, you may see hairline cracks or craze lines. Imagine a pebble hitting your car's windshield: The impact may not destroy it, but a small crack could appear that then becomes a larger crack, until the windshield eventually shatters.
- Do your canines (your eye teeth) look pointy or flat?
- Are there grooves on the outer edges of your tongue? During clenching and grinding, the teeth can 'catch', creating indentations on the sides of the tongue.

I knew we had to not only repair Veena's tooth but also protect the rest of her teeth from further damage. If we didn't, her grinding habit could lead to more chipped teeth or to a deterioration of the supporting bone, which could cause her to eventually lose teeth.

'Yes, there is a piece of tooth missing, Veena. That's the rough spot your tongue is feeling.'

'Oh no!' she said. 'I knew it. Can you fix it?'

'Yes, the rest of the tooth looks okay, so I think a white filling, a composite resin, will hold just fine because it's a small chip. If it doesn't, we may need to consider a stronger material, such as ceramic, but let's start simple.'

'Oh, good,' she said, clearly relieved.

'But we need to discuss what caused your tooth to chip. I don't want you to have any more damaged teeth.'

'Good heavens, nor do I,' she said.

'I see a lot of chipped and cracked teeth in my dental practice these days,' I said. 'It's often due to clenching or grinding.[112] Have you noticed yourself clenching your teeth together or grinding them?'

'I could be,' Veena said. 'I've never thought about it. Sometimes I do wake up with my teeth clamped together.'

'I'm thinking that a lot of the shoulder and neck pain you've been having, and even the headaches, are because you are grinding your teeth.

'Start noticing if that teeth clamping you mentioned when you wake up is happening during the day as well. If it is, put the tip of your tongue to the roof of your mouth and drop your jaw slightly. This position makes it difficult to clench or grind.'

'I'll try,' she said, 'but I don't see how that's going to help when I'm sleeping.'

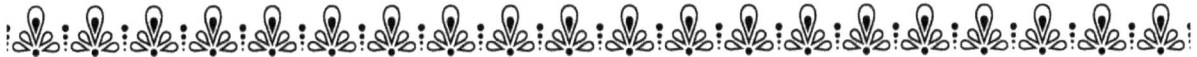

A FINE LINE BETWEEN CLENCHING AND GRINDING

The medical term for Veena's condition is 'bruxism', which is defined as the unconscious act of tightly clenching or grinding the teeth together. Note the word 'unconscious'. This tips us off that awareness alone could begin to change the habit when we are awake.

At night, however, this is not as easy. We can't give that conscious attention to our mouths when we're asleep, and, as with dreaming, we cannot control whether we clench or grind. Disrupting the habit during the day may help reduce the night-time activity, but it rarely solves the problem entirely.

The good news is that there are certain things we CAN do (and should NOT do) to lessen the impacts of this habit. Later in this chapter, I'll share with you some tips based on my own experience as a teeth grinder, my work as a holistic dentist and my knowledge of Ayurveda.

While there's a fine line between clenching and grinding, the signs, symptoms and consequences are basically much the same.

Clenching is when you bite down and squeeze your teeth together very tightly. This can occur when you are awake or asleep. Many of my patients say they've noticed they clench their teeth together when in deep concentration, stressed or angry. Some even tell me they clench while lifting weights at the gym, jogging or driving.

Grinding is when you squeeze your teeth tightly together, as in clenching, but then also move the jaw from side to side. Think of a pestle and mortar. Grinding doesn't necessarily make a sound, so you, or the person lying next to you, may not hear it. And by the way, it's not just adults who clench and grind. Teeth grinding is also common among children.[113]

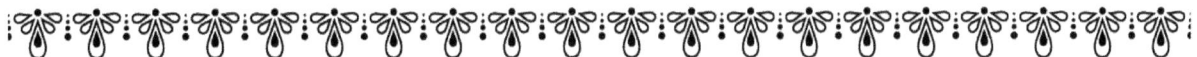

'You're right, Veena, daytime awareness and the tongue trick won't work at night while you're asleep. I recommend that after we repair this chipped tooth, we make you a dental splint that you can wear over your teeth at night. Although this won't stop you from grinding, it will protect your teeth from damage by putting a buffer, a bite plate, in between them.'

'You mean those mouthguards footballers wear? I'm not sure about that,' she said.

'Don't worry,' I said. 'The kind I'll be making for you is thinner than a sports mouthguard. Your lips may bulge out a bit, but you won't look like a footballer.'

'It will take some getting used to, though. We'll work together on easing you in.'

It's not a natural feeling to sleep with a dental appliance in our mouth. Many of my patients spend the first few nights saying, 'I can't do this.' But with time and patience, wearing a dental splint does get easier.

Sharpening Our Teeth for Battle

'Now, let's see if we can find out why you're grinding your teeth, Veena. You said it's been a challenging time.'

'Yes, extremely.'

'Well, I believe this is playing a role in your teeth grinding.'

'I do wish I could relax,' she said. 'It just doesn't seem possible these days.'

This is something many of my patients tell me. Throughout human history, we have always had various stressors or challenges to deal with. These included the threat of animal predators, food scarcity and natural disasters. As a species, we learned to meet these demands fairly well.

Fast forward to this century. The world has changed incredibly rapidly, especially in the past fifty years. High-speed electronic communications and a quicker, more frenetic pace of life are burdening us with an increasing amount of stress unique to today's world. Only fifty years ago, our main methods of communication were quite basic – sending handwritten letters by post and speaking over landline telephones. These days, we can connect with others within a fraction of a second at any time and anywhere in the world.

Our brains, on the other hand, have not evolved as quickly as these new technologies nor have they fully adapted.

Ayurveda recognises that the busyness and stress of modern life can disrupt the balance of our mind, body and spirit. This imbalance can manifest as emotions like anxiety, fear and anger, which can cause us to clench or grind our teeth. In some ancient and esoteric beliefs, teeth grinding is seen as a symbolic act of sharpening teeth in preparation for battle.

From an Ayurvedic perspective, teeth clenching and grinding are signs of an imbalance in the Vata dosha (air) and sometimes in the Pitta dosha (fire).

Dentists worldwide are seeing an increase in teeth grinding.[114] Could it be our body's response to the challenges of these modern times?[115] When we're under stress, our bodies produce the hormone cortisol. Studies have shown that a high level of cortisol directly correlates to the occurrence of bruxism.[116] In other words, when we're under stress, we're more likely to clench and grind our teeth.[117]

I repaired the chip in Veena's tooth and made her a splint. Over the next few weeks, I helped her slowly ease into wearing it.

Initially, I had her wear the splint for an hour or two during the day to allow her mouth and brain to get used to it. The following week, I asked her to try it at night, and in follow-up visits, I adjusted the splint. We continued this process until Veena could comfortably wear her splint through the night.

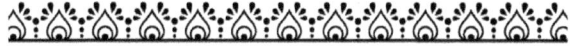

> Dentists worldwide are seeing an increase in teeth grinding. Could it be our body's response to the challenges of these modern times?

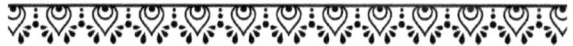

Like Veena, I too grind my teeth, particularly when life is stressful. But unlike her, it was not a chipped tooth that made me aware of this. I had been grinding my teeth so hard without realising it that the nerve in one of my teeth was damaged. The tooth eventually died, and I had to have it extracted. Since then, I've been dedicated to wearing my grinding splint every night. I put it in after I perform my evening oral care.

I say to my patients, 'You're better off spending time with your dental splint than spending time in my chair having your damaged teeth repaired, or worse yet, extracted, as happened to me.'

Because clenching and grinding our teeth at night are mostly unconscious habits exacerbated by stress, the best we can usually do is minimise the damage by taking steps to safeguard our teeth and better manage our stress levels. Fortunately, Ayurvedic wisdom provides a wealth of resources for helping us to slow down and ground ourselves in this fast-paced world.

Beyond Stress: Other Reasons We Clench and Grind Our Teeth

When I took a step back and looked at the bigger picture of Veena's health, I was also aware of other factors that may have been contributing to her teeth grinding habit: her digestive issues, the antidepressant medication she was taking, and the hormonal changes brought on by menopause.

'Another reason you could be grinding, Veena,' I said, 'is because of your leaky gut. Scientists are discovering a link between diseases of the gut and bruxism.'[118]

'How in the world could that be?' Veena said.

'We don't know exactly why, but we're certain that in some way, the jaw is responding to the gut issue.'

These digestive disorders include acid reflux, leaky gut syndrome, gastroesophageal reflux disease (GERD),[119] small intestinal bacterial overgrowth (SIBO), candidiasis and parasites.

'Have you had to change what you eat since your leaky gut diagnosis?' I asked Veena.

'The doctor told me to eat more vegetables and protein, so I've swapped out my morning coffee for a smoothie with protein powder in it and I'm trying to eat healthier all day long.'

'Okay,' I said, 'just make sure you're getting enough calcium, magnesium and vitamin D. Consuming a nutrient-dense diet high in healthy fats, vitamins and minerals should be a priority.'

Calcium and magnesium regulate the contractions of our muscles and support our nervous systems. Magnesium helps our muscles relax, including those around our jaw. It also increases dopamine levels in our brain, which improves our mental state. Vitamin D is another important nutrient. Researchers have found a link between teeth grinding and deficiencies in calcium and vitamin D.[120]

'The antidepressant and the changes in your hormone levels could also be having an effect,' I told Veena. 'If you can, try to avoid caffeine and alcohol.'

Teeth clenching and grinding can be linked to hormonal imbalances (such as menopause), allergies, food intolerances, Parkinson's disease, dementia, attention deficit hyperactivity disorder (ADHD) and epilepsy.

Certain prescription drugs such as antidepressants (SSRIs)[121] and antipsychotics can make people more likely to grind their teeth. The same is true of recreational drugs such as cocaine, MDMA and amphetamines. Even common substances like caffeine and alcohol can have an effect.[122]

'And Veena, this is rather personal, but have you been trying not to cry or get angry?'

'Well, I can't be "losing it" in front of my clients.'

'I understand. Just make sure you let go when you get home. Holding your feelings in can make you want to clench your teeth together.'

Have you ever come across the word *chakra*? Chakra is a Sanskrit word that means wheel or cycle. In Ayurvedic healing, chakras are vital energy centres in the body that must be open and functioning well for us to be healthy and emotionally balanced. The human body has seven chakras. The jaws, along with the rest of the mouth, draw vitality from the throat chakra.

Our feelings and the energy in our throat chakra can become blocked if we are not expressing our truth or living our life purpose, described in Sanskrit as *dharma*. When this flow of energy is obstructed, we tend to bottle up our feelings.

Sometimes we suppress our emotions when what we need to do is cry, or vent our rage. We may hold our breath, clench our jaw and grit our teeth. We 'grin and bear it'. The end result? Our teeth and gums bear the brunt of the impact.

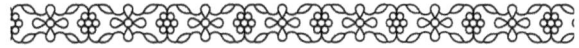

> Ayurvedic wisdom provides a wealth of resources for helping us to slow down and centre ourselves in this fast-paced world.

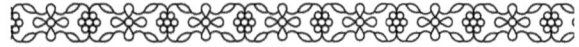

Other Dental Treatments That May Help

When planning dental treatment and the material used to repair teeth, I always take into consideration the fact that the jaw muscles of someone who clenches or grinds their teeth will be more developed and stronger than those of someone who doesn't. Each case must be assessed individually. In the case of Veena, if the chip in her tooth had been larger or in a molar that was under heavy forces, I would have opted for a more durable filling material, such as ceramic.

If Veena's gums had receded to the point where the roots of her teeth were visible, I would have considered placing a white filling over the exposed root surface. This treatment is known as 'bonding'. It protects the tooth from being worn away by brushing and by the acidity in foods and drinks.

If I had discovered an imbalance in Veena's bite that was contributing to her grinding, I would have sought to re-establish balance in her mouth. She might have had a high spot on a filling or crown that was driving an unconscious impulse to grind her teeth. This would be her body's effort to make her teeth fit together better and align with one another. I could adjust the high spot for her quickly and easily by polishing it down.

Or, the uneven bite could be caused by missing teeth, in which case I would recommend filling the gap with a denture, bridge or implant. If her teeth were crowded and affecting her bite, I could suggest orthodontic treatment to align them and restore the bite's natural balance.

I also considered that the imbalance could be coming from her spine. Hard to believe? Consider the skeleton of our body for a moment. Our skull sits at the top of our spinal column. If our spine is not in its natural alignment, then our head won't be in its proper position either. As a result, our jaws and teeth can be out of balance. In such a case, I would refer Veena to an osteopath or a chiropractor.

Enlist a Team to Support You

I believe a holistic approach is a team approach. Just as the mouth isn't a department on its own, so the dentist is often not the only support a person needs to address their dental issues. Sometimes we have to look beyond the mouth to get to the root cause of the problem.

Why not begin creating such a team of your own – a wellness team? On your journey to good health, having others to support you is essential.

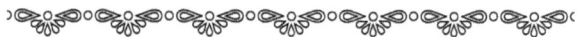

'Veena,' I said, 'I recommend you book yourself a massage once a week to ease your neck and shoulder tension.'

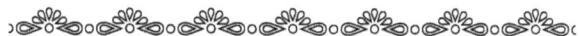

> Why not begin creating such a team of your own – a wellness team? On your journey to good health, having others to support you is essential.

Better Preparation, Better Sleep

'And how is your sleep? You said it's not been good.'

'It's true. My doctor recommended a sleep test because of my weight gain, but it didn't show

I had a sleep disorder. So, I don't know why I'm not sleeping well.'

Many people who clench or grind their teeth while they sleep also have a sleep disorder, such as snoring or sleep apnoea.[123] Until more research is done, we do not know if there is a causal relationship between sleep disorders and teeth grinding, only that there is a correlation.[124]

'It's good to hear you don't have a sleep disorder. Can I ask about your bedtime routine?'

'Oh, I'm so tired from work,' she said, 'that I don't have much energy at the end of the day. I just get into bed and scroll through social media until I nod off.'

'If you can do a few simple things before bed, they will help you relax and sleep better.'

'Sounds like you know something I don't. I would love a good night's sleep.'

As we've seen, stress can have a significant effect on our mouths, manifesting itself in a variety of ways, including teeth clenching and grinding, periodontal disease and even tooth decay. Because bruxism mostly occurs at night, bringing awareness to how we prepare for sleep is important. A restful night's sleep makes just about every other aspect of life much simpler. It is for our physical and mental health, as well as our vitality.

These days, modern science is aware of how important sleep is for overall wellbeing and is immersed in numerous research studies uncovering beneficial sleep habits, such as going to bed at a regular time and avoiding devices and caffeine before bed. These habits are referred to as 'sleep hygiene'.

The importance of sleep has been recognised by Ayurveda for thousands of years. One of the three pillars of wellbeing, sleep, or *Nidra*, is considered as important to health as nutrition and a balanced lifestyle.

We can look to practices that are nurturing and grounding and incorporate them into our night routine of preparing for bed. Earlier, I talked about following the rhythm of the day, Dinacharya. After the sun sets, we can look to another Ayurvedic practice to support us – a night ritual known as *Ratricharya*. (Later, you'll learn more about applying Dinacharya and Ratricharya to your oral care routine.)

I invite you to create your own Ratricharya, choosing the practices that most call you. Make a commitment to introduce three from the list below into your night routine. Your sleep ritual doesn't have to be elaborate. Start simple and build on it slowly so it doesn't become overwhelming – the aim is to relax you, not add stress! It's all about consistency.

We spend almost one-third of our lives sleeping, so why not make it the best? With a few changes in how you prepare for bed, you'll be sleeping better, which will also help you manage your stress and lessen clenching and grinding. You'll be saving your teeth and supporting your overall wellbeing.

Your Prescription for Better Sleep:

1. Avoid food and drink close to bedtime.
   Begin by following the Ayurveda recommendation to make dinner a light meal, the lightest of the day, with at least a couple of hours between drinking and eating, and bedtime. Your kidneys and digestive organs need to rest at night too.

2. Set the scene with some aromatherapy.
   The beauty of nature lies in the many ways in which we can use botanicals to enhance our health and wellbeing.

   By their current popularity, you may think essential oils are a new discovery. In reality, they've been around for thousands of years and were used in many ancient cultures for their aromatic benefits. The oils are extracted from different parts of plants, such as their flowers and leaves, by the process of steam distillation.

In this way, the oils capture the plant's scent and flavour, or 'essence'.

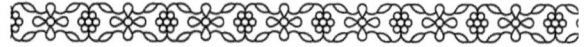

> We spend almost one-third of our lives sleeping, so why not make it the best?

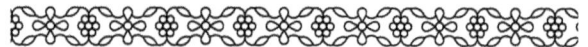

Pure essential oils are not diluted with chemicals or other additives. When used for their scent, we call it aromatherapy. Quite simply, imagine the pleasure you feel when you smell the fragrance of a beautiful flower such as jasmine or a rose. The scents of many essential oils can create feelings of relaxation, which can promote good sleep.

A simple way to enjoy essential oils is to place a few drops in a diffuser or on a tissue, which you can slip inside your pillowcase.

My favourite relaxing oils are lavender, jasmine, sandalwood and rose. Why not get creative and put together a blend of oils that will make your bedroom smell beautiful and help you feel grounded?

3. Consider calming spices and herbs.
   Many spices and herbs from the kitchen have mild sedative properties that can promote a

restful sleep without the addictive potential of pharmaceutical sleeping pills.

Spices like cardamom,[125] turmeric[126] and nutmeg[127] are soothing to the nervous system, helping us feel less anxious and more relaxed. Cinnamon can regulate blood sugar levels during the night, preventing them from fluctuating, which in turn can improve the quality of our sleep.[128] Saffron can influence not only the quality of our sleep but also its duration.[129]

Infuse these spices into your evening tea and drink a cup two hours before bedtime.

In Ayurvedic medicine, herbs have traditionally played an important role in reducing stress and relaxing both mind and body. Ashwaghanda[130] (Withania somnifera), Brahmi[131] (Bacopa monnieri), and Shatavari [132](Asparagus racemosus) are known to relax the nervous system. These herbs, which are referred to as adaptogens in modern medicine, help the body to deal with stress.

(Please note that while these herbs are considered natural, they can be potent. I advise you to consult with a qualified medical practitioner before taking them, particularly if you are pregnant, have any existing medical conditions or are currently taking prescription medications.)

Ayurveda also has a special night-time elixir called Golden Milk. When I was a child, my grandmother would prepare it for me a couple of hours before bedtime to help me relax. Warm milk is considered sleep-inducing in other cultures as well. It contains the hormone melatonin, which supports regular sleep patterns by calming the body and mind.[133] This is why babies usually fall asleep after drinking milk.

Traditional Golden Milk preparations in Ayurveda called for the use of fresh cow's milk. If you are vegan, dairy intolerant or just trying to cut back on dairy, you can create a Golden Milk to suit your needs by substituting almond milk, coconut milk or any other plant-based milk for the cow's milk.

Making a warm Ayurvedic drink in the evening is a beautiful practice that allows you to connect with plant wisdom, relax the mind and nurture more *sattva* (the Sanskrit word for harmony) in preparation for a good night's sleep. By savouring a cup of Golden Milk at the end of a busy day, you can help your body and mind adjust to the gentler, more restorative energy of the evening.

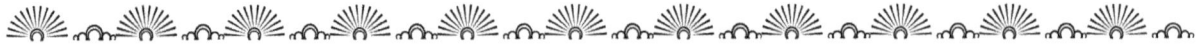

MUMAJI'S GOLDEN MILK

Ingredients

1 cup milk

1/4 tsp. cardamom powder

1/4 tsp. cinnamon powder

1 pinch nutmeg

2 pinches turmeric

2–3 threads saffron (optional)

Warm the milk in a saucepan over low heat until it starts to simmer. Don't let it boil. Remove the saucepan from the heat and let the milk cool slightly. Then whisk in the spices and sweeten as desired with maple syrup or jaggery.

Jaggery is an unrefined natural sugar made from the juices of palm or sugarcane. It has more vitamins and minerals than white sugar. Like ghee, jaggery is a staple in Indian kitchens.

Please don't add honey to your Golden Milk. When heated, honey loses its nutritional value and becomes toxic.[134]

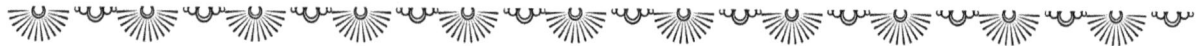

4. Treat yourself to an Ayurvedic self-massage.

A self-massage with warm oil is a nurturing practice that allows us to express love and compassion toward our bodies and souls. In Sanskrit, the single word *sneha* means both oil and love, showing us the connection between the two. Just as receiving love can bring us comfort and warmth, so too can a warm oil massage.

In Ayurveda, this type of massage is known as Abhyanga. Because warm oil is capable of penetrating deeply into the tissues of your body, including your nerve endings, it's ideal for calming the body and mind before sleep and relieving insomnia. While traditional Ayurvedic texts recommend performing Abhyanga first thing in the morning, I suggest adapting this practice to the evening to help you relax before bedtime.

The primary dosha linked with anxiety,

restlessness and disturbed sleep is Vata, whose airy, ethereal aspects are balanced and grounded by the oil.

In addition to producing a sense of grounding and relaxation, a daily oil massage can improve your health in so many ways, from better circulation and detoxification to softer skin and more supple joints.

You can do it in three simple steps.

Step 1: Choose an oil.

Your skin is your largest organ, and whatever you put on it is absorbed directly into your body. For this reason, choose the best quality oil you can find, preferably organic and extra-virgin.

If you resonate with Vata traits or live in a cooler climate, use black sesame oil for its warming quality. Coconut oil is more cooling and suited for those with Pitta traits or those living in a warmer climate. Due to their heavier nature, Kapha types should use a lighter oil such as safflower to balance the heaviness. If you're unsure which dosha is dominant in you, find out by taking the Ayurveda Dosha Quiz in Appendix A.

Mahanarayan Thailam is an Ayurvedic oil blend infused with a combination of herbs especially good for soothing sore muscles and lubricating joints. This oil can be applied to the area around the jaw muscles and the TMJ, a perfect elixir for the teeth grinder. Just add three to four drops to your primary massage oil.

Step 2: Choose which massage you'd like to do.

To receive the full benefits of an Ayurvedic self-massage, it's best to do one every night if possible or at least two to three times a week. Just make sure at least two hours have passed since you last ate.

If you don't have time for a whole-body massage, consider doing a head massage (Shiro Abhyanga) or a foot massage (Pada Abhyanga)[135] following the same procedure as in the full-body massage, but focusing on only your head or feet. Shiro Abhyanga has been shown by modern science to help with insomnia and promote sound sleep.

When I was a child, my grandmother would seat me on the floor in front of her chair and massage my head with sesame oil. I always slept so well after that. She did it with so much love.

If you don't have or want to use oil, then warm, moist heat will do. Simply place a facecloth in hot water and wring it out. Press the warm, wet towel around your jaw, neck and shoulder muscles, massaging gently.

Step 3: Do the massage.

To warm the oil, pour half a cup into a bowl and place the bowl inside a larger container of simmering water. Allow the oil to heat for ten to fifteen minutes until it is warm to the touch.

You may want to add a couple of drops of Mahanarayan Thailam or a soothing essential oil to the mix.

Stand on a large towel. Abhyanga is best done in the bathroom. If you need to sit, use a small stool or the edge of the bathtub.

To begin, apply oil to your feet and massage it in, using the fingertips of both hands, applying moderate pressure and moving your hands in firm circular motions.

Carry out that same motion all the way up the legs. After that, move on to your hands, arms, stomach, chest and back, then your face, neck and shoulders, and finally your head. If you clench or grind your teeth, devote extra attention to massaging the warm oil around your ears, TMJs, jaw muscles and forehead, including your third eye, located between and slightly above your eyebrows.

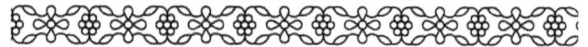

Allow the oil to remain on your skin for ten to twenty minutes so it can work its way into the deeper layers. Some of my patients make use of this time to perform their oral care ritual in preparation for bed.

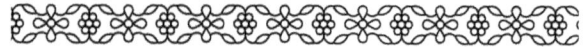

> If you clench or grind your teeth, devote extra attention to massaging the warm oil around your ears, TMJs, jaw muscles and forehead, including your third eye, located between and slightly above your eyebrows.

When the time is up, wipe off any excess oil with an old towel or sarong. Rinse off briefly with a warm shower and gently pat your skin dry so that it retains the moisture from the oil.

5. Declutter your mind.

At least one hour before going to bed, tune out from the busyness of the day and tune in to the quieter energy of the evening. Although it may be tempting to scroll through the news and social media feeds, we need to give our nervous system the time and space to unwind before bed. Disconnect from your digital devices, television and social media. Otherwise, you will be trying to sleep while you are wired.

Instead, tune into the serene sounds of nature or gentle music designed for meditation. These sound frequencies resemble those found in the natural world and have the ability to influence our internal systems, such as blood pressure, heart rate, anxiety levels and even digestion. One such set of frequencies is known as Solfeggio, which is made up of specific tones believed to have ancient origins in both Western Christianity and Eastern religions. They've been recited by Gregorian monks and can also be found in Sanskrit chants from India.

You can find a wide range of Solfeggio sounds by simply searching the internet.

Chanting a mantra is another way to calm the mind. Mantras are words or phrases that are spoken or sung in certain religious and spiritual traditions, such as Buddhism and Hinduism, as a means of bringing the mind into a state of inner stillness and focus. The word *mantra* comes from a combination of two Sanskrit words that mean 'a tool to stabilise the mind'. Mantras are believed to possess a strong spiritual energy due to the powerful vibrations created by their sound. Once you find a mantra that resonates with you, simply close your eyes and repeat the chosen word or phrase until you feel centered and relaxed. Remember, your mantra can be as simple as you like and doesn't have to be in Sanskrit.

A Vedic mantra I find comforting to chant before bed is *Aum shanti, shanti, shanti*, which translates as 'peace, peace, peace'. This mantra invokes peace to the heavens, to all sentient beings on the earth and to oneself.

To declutter our minds and promote emotional wellbeing, Ayurveda advises us to examine our emotions regularly. Just as we digest and process our food, we should also digest and process our emotions on a daily basis. This can be as simple as journalling or carrying out an emotions inventory at night. Take a few minutes to reflect: How did you feel throughout the day? What went well and what's bothering you? Is there anything you need to do to 'put things right?' How would you like to feel? What will you do differently tomorrow to enable you to feel that way?

6. Get heavy with a weighted blanket.

Weighted blankets have become increasingly popular for helping with anxiety and insomnia. These blankets are heavier than regular blankets, usually weighing around ten to twelve kg (twenty-two to twenty-six pounds), with lighter options available for children.

According to modern research, the pressure exerted by a weighted blanket can have a calming effect on the nervous system, similar to the benefits of a massage. This is why babies are soothed when they are swaddled, that is, wrapped tightly in a cloth.

This pressure stimulates the release of serotonin, oxytocin and melatonin[136] in the brain, important hormones for promoting relaxation and sleep.[137]

From an Ayurvedic perspective, a weighted blanket is perfect for grounding the flighty qualities of Vata dosha. I offer weighted blankets to my anxious patients at Anokhi Dental.

Now that I've given you my top six tips for a restful night, choose the one that most appeals to you and begin.

Veena started by turning her iPad off an hour before bed. She also booked herself a remedial massage and noticed the benefits almost immediately – her neck and shoulders felt less tense, and she experienced fewer headaches.

For emotional support, Veena started to see a therapist to process her grief. I have no doubt that talking it out is helping her release the constricted energy in her jaws. She has also stepped completely out of her comfort zone and attended a few meditation retreats, which, to her surprise, she has enjoyed.

Although Veena still has stressors in her life, as we all do, she now has ways to better manage that stress. And she can sleep easier at night knowing her teeth are protected by her dental splint.

She thanked me for getting her started on the road to healing and good health. And all because of a chipped tooth!

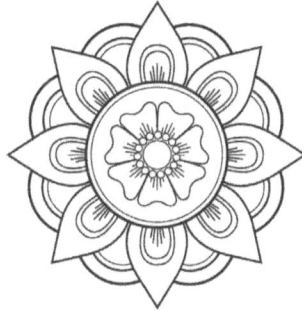

PART 3

Your New Relationship With Your Mouth

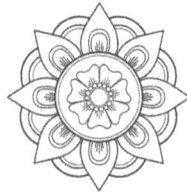

CHAPTER 6

FROM MUNDANE TO ENJOYABLE

Turn Your Daily Dental Routine into a Beautiful, Nourishing Ritual

Jaya, twenty, is visiting my clinic for the first time for a routine check-up and teeth cleaning. She's just moved from New York to Sydney to study piano at the Australian Institute of Music. Because Jaya grew up with a mother devoted to natural health, she has always had a holistic dentist and chose Anokhi Dental for that reason.

Helping young people learn how to prevent dental issues like those experienced by Julian, Ruby and Veena is a rewarding part of my career.

'Simply put,' I tell them, 'less is more. I want us to focus on prevention.'

As I looked over Jaya's medical history, I saw she had no health issues and wasn't taking any medications, although she did take some vitamins from time to time.

'Music school is pretty demanding,' she told me. 'And moving to a new country has been exciting but tiring. I'm now feeling settled enough to get back into the routine of regular dental check-ups.

'I'm embarrassed to admit, though, that in the past couple of months, I haven't been great with my dental care. I try to floss before bed when my hands aren't too sore from playing the piano.'

'Okay, let's see if we can put together an easy routine for you. It doesn't have to take long, just three or four minutes. It can be simple.'

'It has to be!' she said. 'My mornings are a

rush because I have to be at the Conservatory by 7:30. I'm also there late a few nights a week.'

'What do you do when you wake up?'

'First, I have a hot lemon water drink. Then I eat some breakfast and brush my teeth before heading out.'

'Okay, the first thing I want you to do when you wake up, Jaya, is clean your mouth, within the first three minutes. This is one of the most important self-care practices of the day.

'At night, when we're sleeping, our mouth is less active than during the day. We don't make as much saliva, which makes our mouth drier. In a dry environment, dead cells, bacteria and toxins build up, particularly on the tongue, gums and teeth.

'If you don't clean your mouth as soon as you wake up, but instead start eating and drinking, you'll end up swallowing whatever has accumulated in your mouth overnight. It's like drinking water from a dirty, stagnant pond.'

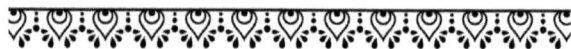

Jaya wrinkled her nose.

'You don't want to be sending harmful bacteria and toxins back down into your stomach and ultimately into your entire body.'

'That sounds awful,' Jaya said. 'From now on, I'll brush first thing.'

'Actually,' I said, 'there's one thing you can do

before you brush your teeth. I'll go over that after your check-up.'

'Okay, sounds good.'

'My other concern is your lemon water drink,' I said. 'Although it's good for you, it's quite acidic, just like apple cider vinegar and kombucha. The acid can soften the surface of your teeth. If you eat or brush straight after the drink, you'll be scraping off that softened enamel, which can eventually lead to exposed dentine and tooth sensitivity. It can also make your teeth look more yellow over time.'

'I don't want that,' Jaya said, shaking her head.

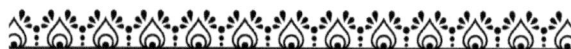

> 'If you don't clean your mouth as soon as you wake up, but instead go straight to eating and drinking, you'll end up swallowing whatever has accumulated in your mouth overnight. It's like drinking water from a dirty, stagnant pond.'

'I suggest waiting one hour after drinking the lemon water before brushing your teeth or eating. This gives your saliva time to remineralise your teeth. I also recommend drinking the lemon water through a bamboo straw and rinsing your mouth with room temperature water as soon as you're done.'

'Wow, I didn't know all that. Thank you.'

As I looked in Jaya's mouth, I saw that her teeth and gums were healthy.

'Okay, Jaya, all is good. Now, let's talk about your routine. Here's what I want you to do.'

Greeting the Day: Your Morning Ritual

To reap the most benefits, it's important to follow a specific sequence when cleaning your mouth. In the morning, I recommend four simple steps in the following order:

1. Look at your tongue.
2. Clean your teeth.
3. Clean your tongue.
4. Oil pull.

Why is it important to follow this order? There are two main reasons: First, if you brush your teeth and floss *after* cleaning your tongue, you risk dislodging plaque, which may then land on your freshly cleaned tongue. Second, if you swish with an oil-based mouthwash after you've

cleaned your teeth, gums and tongue, your mouth will receive the full benefits of the oil. While I have encountered several differing opinions about when to oil pull, some suggesting it be done before cleaning the teeth and tongue, as a dentist, I recommend doing it last. Do whatever you feel most comfortable with, but please, do oil pull.

The mouth is not only one of the most used parts of the body but also one of the most sensitive. We eat and drink with it, speak and sing with it, and smile and kiss with it. For some of us, it's what we breathe through. Our mouth enables us to communicate with the outer world and nourish our inner world, fulfilling two fundamental needs essential to our human existence.

We can acknowledge and honour the important role played by the mouth in our overall health by cultivating a personalised dental routine. This transformative practice can elevate an everyday 'must-do' into a nurturing self-care ritual, something you look forward to and enjoy.

By embracing this practice, you'll be honouring the Ayurvedic tradition of Dinacharya – to follow 'the knowledge of the day'.

You can craft your very own 'Oral Dinacharya', a personal ritual that addresses the particular needs of your unique mouth. How will you care for your teeth and gums? Which toothpaste will you use? What type of mouthwash?

Embarking on a new routine can often feel daunting. With each repetition, however, it becomes easier, eventually becoming second nature. The process of transforming a novel behaviour into a habit usually takes around twenty-one days. With this knowledge, we can practise patience and be gentle with ourselves as we integrate these actions into our lives.

Maintaining a day-to-day routine will help you avoid costly and invasive dental procedures in the future. Imagine taking care of your car: While it's important to have it serviced by a mechanic once or twice a year, how you treat and maintain it the rest of the time is what determines its performance and how long it will last. This is also true for how we take care of our mouth.

Let's get started.

Ritual Step 1: Look at your tongue.

'It's a good habit to check your tongue from time to time,' I told Jaya. 'It doesn't have to be every day, but when you do, do it before cleaning your mouth. Your tongue can provide insights into your overall health and wellbeing.'

'Okay,' she said, 'I had no idea.'

'You've heard the expression about the eyes being the window to the soul?'

'Yes,' she said.

'Well, the mouth, especially the tongue, is the window into our health, from the inside out. When I looked at your tongue today, it looked healthy.'

In the realms of ancient Indian and Chinese medicine, the tongue is a valuable and non-invasive diagnostic tool. If you were to visit one of these practitioners, they would probably look at your tongue as part of their examination.

You can adopt these traditional practices by checking your own tongue in the mirror. (Please note that a self-examination should not be regarded as a substitute for diagnosis and appropriate treatment from a qualified medical practitioner.)

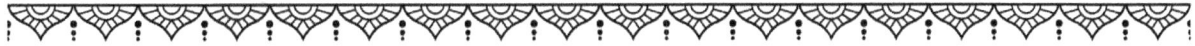

WHAT IS YOUR TONGUE TELLING YOU?

Do you notice a coating? – Is there a sticky film on your tongue, similar to the plaque you might feel on your teeth? If so, you may be experiencing issues with digestion, which can result in an accumulation of Ama within the body. Check where the coating appears. If it's on the back of your tongue, it's possible you have toxins in your gut, which is common given our modern eating habits.

Can you see teeth marks? – Do the sides of your tongue have any indentations or notches? If so, you may not be absorbing nutrients properly and/ or you may be grinding your teeth.

Malabsorption can occur when we eat foods that aren't right for us or when our digestion is sluggish. It can lead to inflammation or imbalances in the gut.

Are there any cracks? – If you have small cracks or fissures on your tongue, you are most likely under stress. You may be experiencing anxiety, fear or insomnia.

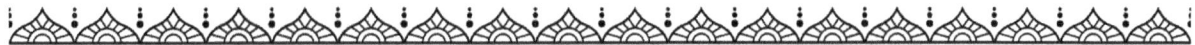

Ritual Step 2: Clean your teeth.

'After you look at your tongue,' I told Jaya, 'go on to cleaning your teeth. I'm glad to hear that you try to brush morning and night. Plaque builds up on our teeth around the clock.

'If you could brush after every meal, that would be even better because you'd be removing the food particles that harmful bacteria feed on. I know it's not easy with your schedule.

'What kind of toothbrush do you use?'

'Just the regular plastic ones I get at the grocery store.'

'Have you heard of bamboo toothbrushes?' I asked.

'I may have, but I haven't actually seen one.'

Which Toothbrush Should You Use?

These days we have so many choices when choosing a toothbrush. It can be quite confusing.

As an earth-friendly alternative to plastic, I recommend bamboo toothbrushes to my patients. Bamboo is hard to beat in terms of sustainability: It grows quickly without the need for chemical fertilisers or pesticides. It's also biodegradable, unlike plastic, which sits in landfills for at least five hundred years before breaking down. Our planet already has too much plastic. We don't need any more.

Choose a toothbrush with soft, wavy bristles long enough to bend into all the crevices in your mouth. A hard brush with short, stiff bristles can be abrasive on the teeth and gums, much like rough sandpaper on polished wood.

I am often asked by my patients if an electric toothbrush is better than a manual one. From my experience as a dentist, looking into thousands of mouths over the years, I can honestly say I don't think so. I've seen poor oral hygiene in patients who use an electric toothbrush and excellent cleaning in patients who use a manual one. It's all about consistency and technique, which I'll tell you about in a moment.

And really, do we need another gadget to rely on? In the event that our electric toothbrush stopped working, we would find ourselves in a predicament because our routine had become so dependent on it.

Another perspective to consider in the electric-vs-manual toothbrush debate is to ask ourselves if we really want more electricity in our lives. Despite our efforts to unwind from the demands of modern life through practices like yoga, meditation and conscious breathing, we often find ourselves surrounded by technology that has the opposite effect. Plugging in an electronic device and whizzing through our teeth cleaning as if it were a task to simply zip through can appear to be convenient and time-saving, but what we really need in this fast-paced world is to slow down. By embracing a mindful approach to our daily practices, we can transform them into meaningful and enriching experiences.

One scenario where I do feel an electric toothbrush can be helpful is when someone has difficulty gripping and manoeuvring a toothbrush, perhaps due to arthritis in the hands or an injury.

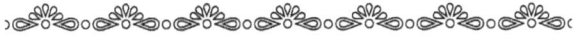

> By embracing a mindful approach to our daily practices, we can transform them into meaningful and enriching experiences.

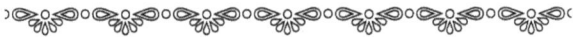

Manual or electric toothbrush aside, the key to good brushing is the *way* in which you brush. I recommend small circular motions over all the surfaces of each tooth – top, front, back and sides – with a focus around the gum line, where the tooth and gum meet, because this is where the majority of germs and plaque accumulate.

'To make it fun,' I told Jaya, 'you might try brushing your teeth with your non-dominant hand. Are you right-handed?'

'I am,' she said. 'So, you're saying I should try brushing with my left hand?' Jaya smiled. 'Like playing the bass clef on the piano.'

I laughed. 'Yes, exactly. The idea is to try something different, something that isn't second nature. Modern science shows that novel activities can help us develop new neural pathways in our brain. Although it hasn't been specifically proven that brushing with the opposite hand is one of those activities, it can be a way to slow down and be more mindful of what we're doing.'

'That's so interesting,' she said. 'Maybe it will improve my piano playing. I'm going to try it.'

'Great,' I said.

'It's interesting that we don't make brushing our teeth a priority or do it more often. Did you know that people in ancient cultures cleaned their teeth several times throughout the day?'

Jaya shook her head.

'People in India, the Egyptians, the Babylonians, the Greeks, and the Africans would chew on twigs from aromatic herbs and kept the twigs in their mouths throughout the day.'[138]

The Traditional Chewing Stick

In ancient India, chewing on certain bitter herbal sticks used to be the traditional way of cleaning the teeth. These sticks were known to reduce the buildup of plaque and stimulate saliva production, both important for a healthy mouth.

Skip ahead a few thousand years and you'll find modern research has confirmed this ancient knowledge: Traditional chewing sticks offer many benefits for the mouth.[139]

Even if we're living in the twenty-first century, we can tap into the oral care practices of earlier times. It's still possible to purchase chewing sticks, referred to as *Datoon* in Sanskrit. These sticks include liquorice root (Glycyrrhiza glabra), neem (Azadirachta indica), babool (Acacia arabica) and miswak (Salvadora persica).

They all have natural antimicrobial properties that stop the growth of harmful oral bacteria. The action of chewing on the sticks can also help dislodge food and stimulate saliva production, which helps cleanse the mouth.

In the humble Datoon stick, ancient Indians had an all-in-one tool for complete oral care: a stick that could mechanically clean like a toothbrush, a tool to clean around and in between the teeth and a mouthwash from the stick's medicinal juices. An ingenious one-stop shop that was ahead of its time and a fun way for us to connect to an ancient Ayurvedic tradition.

Chewing on herbal sticks can help reduce plaque build-up, prevent decay and combat bad breath. It can even revitalise the taste senses. That said, considering our modern lifestyle choices, stress and eating habits, I still recommend an oral care routine that includes brushing, flossing and regular dental check-ups.

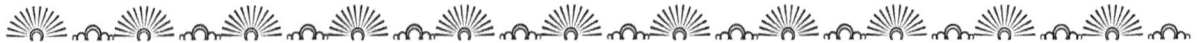

HOW TO USE A CHEWING STICK

Rinse the twig with water, then chew on one end of it until the juices emerge. Swish those juices around in your mouth and spit them out after 10–20 seconds.

Now, gently brush your teeth with the exposed 'bristles', taking care not to hurt your gums. You can also use the twig to gently clean between the teeth, much like a toothpick. Feel free to give the twig another round of chewing, spit out the juice and get back to brushing.

After you've finished brushing, rinse your mouth with water, cut off the frayed end of the twig and keep the stick for future use.

Remember, chewing on herbal sticks does not replace your toothbrush and floss. It is only an adjunct to good oral care.

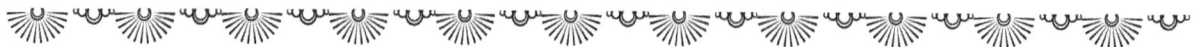

Should You Brush Your Gums If They're Receding?

Some of my patients with receding gums believe they're making their situation worse by brushing near their gums. As a result, they either reduce the amount of time they brush or stop brushing altogether.

If you have receding gums, you should still brush at the junction of your gums and teeth, though carefully. Why? Because bacteria and inflammation will build up, which can lead to more gum recession and gum disease. I recommend brushing your teeth using a soft-bristled toothbrush with small circular motions and a light touch.

How to Care for Your Toothbrush

Please, never share a toothbrush with someone else, no matter how much you love them. Treat your toothbrush like a password.

Where you store it is also important. Be mindful to keep your toothbrush away from the toilet in an upright position so that it can air dry, preferably in a cabinet away from dust and other airborne particles. Or place it on a windowsill that receives direct sunlight, where the sun's rays will both dry and sterilise your toothbrush.

You could also use two toothbrushes and alternate between them, allowing each one to dry in between uses.

When Should You Change Your Toothbrush?

We may think keeping and using a toothbrush for an extended time is economical and kind to the planet. It's important, however, to replace it on a regular basis.

As a general rule, I recommend a new toothbrush every three months, or sooner if:

- the bristles start to fray
- you've been sick
- you've dropped your toothbrush on the floor
- somebody else has used it by mistake.

Which Toothpaste Should You Use?

'Now,' I said to Jaya, 'let's talk about your toothpaste. What are you using?'

'I usually buy a whitening one from the supermarket because I want my smile to look good, especially if I have a performance.'

Like Jaya, at any given time, you may have chosen a specific toothpaste based on claims like whitening teeth or freshening breath.

These are all perfectly reasonable desires, but they're often achieved with ingredients that should not be in our mouths.

'I'd like you to switch to a natural toothpaste,' I told Jaya. 'You'll be avoiding chemicals that can be harmful to your mouth and your body.'

'I didn't know toothpastes had anything bad in them,' she said. 'They all claim to do great things for your teeth.'

'Yes, the problem is that the majority of dental care products were originally formulated over a century ago by detergent manufacturers. Their aim was to eradicate every microbe in sight.

'But now we know that when we destroy *all* bacteria, we disrupt the delicate balance of the oral microbiome.'

Wiping out all the bacteria in the mouth is comparable to what happens in our gut when we take a course of antibiotics. Both harmful and beneficial bacteria are eliminated. This is why it's so important to repopulate the gut with good bacteria by taking probiotics in the form of supplements or fermented foods.

'And, Jaya, harsh ingredients found in oral care products can spread from your mouth to other parts of your body. Let me show you how that happens.'

I handed her a mirror.

'Put your tongue to the roof of your mouth and look in the mirror,' I said. 'Do you see all those blood vessels? They give the mouth an incredibly rich blood supply.

'That means that whatever is in our mouth can be absorbed very quickly into the bloodstream.'

Medical professionals are aware that when a patient experiences chest pain due to reduced blood supply to the heart, a condition known as angina, immediate relief can be provided by spraying a medication under their tongue. It reaches the heart within a fraction of a second. Similarly, homeopathic drops are placed under the tongue for the same purpose of rapid absorption and effectiveness.

'That's amazing,' Jaya said. 'I never thought about my mouth that way, that it's connected to my body.'

'We absorb ninety per cent of whatever comes into contact with our mouth, so we do *not* want to place a toxic substance there. If it's in your mouth, it's in your body.'

A Word about Ingredients

The boom in the health and wellness industry, coupled with the vast amount of information available on the internet, has helped us start to see that many mainstream, mass-manufactured products do not truly support our health. They often contain synthetic chemicals and toxic ingredients that can harm us and the environment. This extends to many of the toothpastes and mouthwashes you'll find on the market.

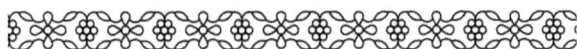

> 'We absorb ninety per cent of whatever comes into contact with our mouth, so we do not want to place a toxic substance there. If it's in your mouth, it's in your body.'

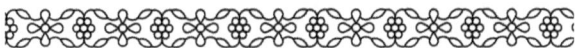

Triclosan, a chemical commonly found in toothpastes, has been associated with hormone disruption, and its use has been banned in many countries.

Another harmful ingredient is sodium lauryl sulphate, a foaming agent used in toothpastes and mouthwashes. Research has shown that this chemical can contribute to an increased occurrence of mouth ulcers in people who are prone to them.[140]

So just as you are mindful about what food you put in your mouth and body, also be mindful of what is in your oral care products.

Please avoid these ingredients:

- Alcohol
- Fluoride
- Foaming agents such as Sodium lauryl sulphate (SLS), Diethanolamine (DEA) and Propylene glycol
- Artificial flavours, colours (such as titanium dioxide) and sweeteners (sorbitol, saccharin and aspartame)
- Triclosan
- Carrageenan
- Parabens

To steer clear of these harmful ingredients, we can turn to nature to support our wellbeing, as our ancestors did. The earth generously provides us with minerals, plants and fruits, many of which can be beneficial for dental health.

The ingredients and recipes I recommend draw on that wisdom. When you're finished reading, you'll know what to look for in any toothpaste or mouthwash you might purchase and also what natural, healthier alternatives you can use instead.

You may even be inspired to get creative and make your own oral care products based on the unique needs of your mouth and infused with the flavours and qualities that most appeal to you. Voila! Your very own personal dental care system.

So, what exactly should you look for when choosing a toothpaste? Yes, it should be as natural as possible, but the word 'natural' is used frequently these days and can be interpreted in several different ways. Even though they claim to be natural, certain toothpastes on the market do contain at least one of the potentially harmful chemicals I've listed above.

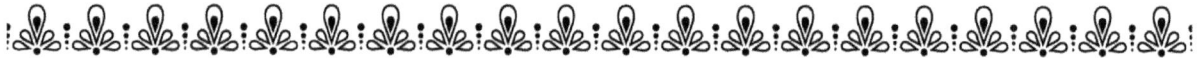

WHAT YOUR MOUTH IS ASKING FOR

Your mouth wants ingredients that are:

- naturally antibacterial and target only the harmful bacteria, while leaving the helpful bacteria in place to continue their good work (many of the spices and herbs in Ayurvedic medicine – clove, cinnamon, liquorice, neem and fennel, for example – are antibacterial with the added bonus of naturally freshening the breath)

- alkalising to reduce acidity and increase alkalinity for a healthy, balanced oral microbiome (bentonite clay is one such ingredient)
- teeth strengthening by offering minerals that can help remineralise and repair them (hydroxyapatite is powerful in this role).

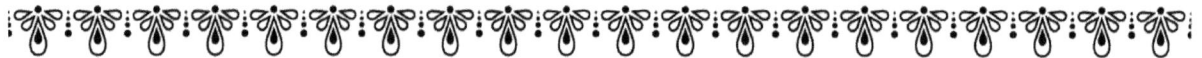

The Proper Way to Clean Between Your Teeth

Even if you clean your teeth thoroughly, plaque and bacteria can still build up in the gaps between them, making this a perfect spot for decay to develop. This is why it's important to clean in between your teeth every day.

'You mentioned that you floss your teeth at night,' I said to Jaya. 'Do you hear a "click" when you do that?'

'Yes,' she said.

'That's good. When you hear a "click" while flossing, it means your teeth are sitting tightly next to each other and flossing may be enough to clean between them.

'If you don't hear a "click" or if the floss feels loose as it passes through, you could have larger spaces between your teeth. In this case, something thicker than floss, like an interdental brush might be more effective.'

The term 'inter-dental' literally translates to 'between the teeth'. Interdental brushes are small, thin brushes with fine bristles that can glide between teeth to remove plaque, food particles and debris.

They're like miniature versions of the brushes used to clean baby bottles and are available in different sizes. And just like toothbrushes, interdental brushes are now being made with bamboo handles, which is, of course, preferable to plastic.

Interdental brushes are not only useful for cleaning larger gaps between the teeth but also around dental appliances such as orthodontic braces, bridgework and dental implants.

While I may not be enthusiastic about electronic gadgets, I occasionally recommend the use of a water flosser to clean around dental appliances or deep gum pockets. Also known as an oral irrigator, the flosser emits a high-pressure, pulsating stream of water to flush out food particles, plaque and bacteria from the spaces between the teeth and the gum pockets.

Ritual Step 3: Clean your tongue.

'There are a couple of things I'd like you to add to your routine, Jaya, that won't take long. After you clean your teeth, I want you to clean your tongue, especially in the morning.'

'I sometimes run my toothbrush over my tongue if it feels furry,' she said.

'I'd prefer you use a tongue scraper, which is specifically designed to clean the tongue. A toothbrush, as its name implies, is made for cleaning teeth. If you use your toothbrush to clean your tongue, you run the risk of transferring bacteria from your teeth to your tongue and vice versa. You don't want to spread bacteria around different parts of your mouth any more than you would want a friend to use your toothbrush.'

When you think of your dental hygiene routine, does it include cleaning your tongue?

Considering how much space it takes up in the mouth, tongue hygiene should be up there with brushing and flossing. It's the hardest worker in the mouth, allowing us to taste and enjoy our food. It moves food around in our mouth when we're chewing and enables us to swallow and speak.

Ayurvedic medicine recognises the interconnectedness of the tongue, digestive health and overall health. It understands that our digestive organs process food throughout the day and along the way accumulate Ama.

During the night while we sleep, our body undergoes natural detoxification and elimination processes. The toxins and bacteria released migrate up the mucous lining of the gut into the mouth, settling as a coating on the tongue.

The state of our digestive health can be determined not only by the appearance of our tongue, as I described earlier, but also by the smell of our breath. A coating on the tongue and bad breath first thing in the morning are signs of Ama, toxic substances that our bodies are working hard to get rid of. According to Ayurveda, the build-up of Ama is believed to be the underlying cause of various diseases.

The Ayurvedic practice of daily tongue cleaning known as *Jihva Prakshalana* is a quick, easy way to remove Ama and helps balance the oral microbiome, supporting overall health and immunity.

Other benefits include fresher breath, better digestion and an improved sense of taste. When our sense of taste improves, we savour our food more. We feel satisfied more quickly and are less likely to overeat.

Research also tells us that cleaning the tongue supports the bacteria that make a substance called nitric oxide, which is needed for maintaining stable blood pressure and preventing sexual dysfunction.[141]

When I was growing up, nobody in my family would have dreamed of starting the day without cleaning their tongue first thing in the morning. It's a daily practice in India and one just as important as cleaning the teeth.

'Okay,' Jaya said, 'but I have no idea how to do it.'

'That's all right. It's very easy. Let me show you.'

HOW TO CLEAN YOUR TONGUE

I suggest purchasing a copper tongue cleaner as it is naturally antibacterial. Alternatively, silver or stainless steel tongue cleaners are also fine, while plastic ones should be avoided.

I don't recommend the use of tongue cleaners for children under the age of five. If you do see a coating on your child's tongue, I suggest using the back of a teaspoon to clean it off, which will be gentler.

To perform tongue cleaning, follow these steps:

1. Extend your tongue out of your mouth, allowing it to protrude comfortably.
2. Hold the two ends of the tongue cleaner in both hands.
3. With a gentle, yet steady pressure, glide the tongue cleaner from the middle to the front of your tongue. If you gag, you are placing the cleaner too far back, and if your tongue bleeds, you are scraping too hard.
4. Repeat this process three times down the middle of the tongue and three times on either side.
5. After each stroke, rinse the tongue cleaner to remove any accumulated debris.

In less than ten seconds your tongue is clean.

After using your tongue cleaner, rinse it and store it with your toothbrush. This way you'll remember to use it after brushing.

Over time, a copper tongue cleaner may develop tarnish. While this tarnish isn't harmful to your mouth, it can be removed by rubbing it with a lemon wedge and sea salt. This will restore your tongue cleaner to its original shine.

You're now ready for the final step of your oral care ritual.

Ritual Step 4: Oil pull.

'The last step I'd like you to take, Jaya, is to do something called oil pulling.'

'Oh, yes, I've seen something about that on Instagram, but I don't know much about it.'

'Oil pulling is an Ayurvedic practice that involves swishing oil in the mouth to cleanse it. The ancient texts recommend holding the oil in the mouth for ten to twenty minutes, but it doesn't have to be that long. I do my oil pulling while I make my bed every morning, which makes it easy to remember.'

In Sanskrit, oil pulling is called both *gandusha*, the practice of holding liquid in the mouth and *kavala*, which is more like swishing and gargling as you would a mouthwash.

'Do you have something you do every day that could be a good time to oil pull?' I asked Jaya.

'Well, I like to play a five-minute piece I'm working on as a warm-up before I leave for school. I could do it then.'

'Perfect,' I said.

Exactly how oil pulling works isn't fully understood, and scientific research on the topic is limited. It is thought that when oil is swished in the mouth, it creates a pulling or dragging effect that helps dislodge bacteria, plaque and other debris from the teeth and gums. The oil also attracts and binds oil-soluble toxins in the mouth, similar to how soap pulls dirt from clothes and dishes. The toxins are then expelled from the body when the oil is spat out.

Why Oil Pulling is Beneficial in More Ways than One

Whatever the reason oil pulling works, it does. Research has shown that swishing with oil in the mouth for ten to twenty minutes a day can decrease the amount of bacteria[142] that lead to bad breath, gum disease and tooth decay.[143] Oil pulling also reduces plaque and stimulates saliva production.[144] Saliva contains enzymes, antibodies and minerals essential for a healthy mouth. These enzymes absorb toxins, which also helps to purify the body. According to Ayurveda, removing toxins from the mouth can help remove toxins from other parts of the body as well.[145]

When the oil is in the mouth, it coats the teeth and gums, acting as a protective barrier against bacteria adhering to and penetrating them. Your gums will be nourished and moisturised.

One of the best things about cleansing the mouth with an oil or oil-based mouthwash is that it doesn't strip the mouth of beneficial bacteria the way commercial mouthwashes containing alcohol and antiseptic chemicals do.

'I'm keen to try this,' Jaya said.

'Great!' I said. 'Go ahead and start small, three or four minutes while you're playing that short piece at the piano. You can always build up the time. It doesn't matter if you work up to only five minutes or ten. Either way, it's fine.

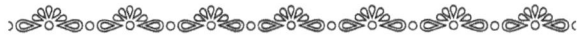

> Research has shown that swishing with oil in the mouth for ten to twenty minutes a day can decrease the amount of bacteria that lead to bad breath, gum disease and tooth decay.

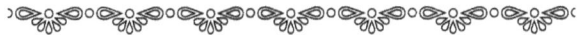

'You know, we're not living in Ancient India five thousand years ago where life was a lot simpler and we had more time. Just do what you can.

'I'm sure that once you start to enjoy how clean your mouth feels after oil pulling,' I said, 'you won't want to miss a day. My patients often tell me, "Wow, my mouth and breath feel so much fresher." Some of them even say their teeth look whiter.'

'But I don't know where to start,' Jaya said. 'I mean, which oil do I use?'

'Many people like coconut oil, which has a milder flavour than the traditionally used sesame oil. Studies have found either oil is effective.'[146]

'Oh, I love the taste of coconut oil. I use it for cooking.'

Which Oil is Best?

Although the properties of different oils are unique, they all work in the same way. Traditionally, sesame oil was used for oil pulling; its taste, however, may not be appealing to everyone. More popular these days is coconut oil for its breath-freshening properties, ability to combat bacteria and teeth-whitening effects.

Another oil that works well for oil pulling, although not as well known, is ghee, which you learned about in terms of cavity prevention. Ghee contains Omega-3 fatty acids and vitamin A, which help soothe the gums, promote healing and maintain a healthy mouth lining.

Each oil – sesame, coconut or ghee – can be used on its own. Or, you could make your own medicated oil, a common practice in Ayurveda, by adding the herbs and spices appropriate for your particular dental needs.

If you suffer from dry mouth, for example, add papaya seed oil[147] or ginger oil to your base oil. Both encourage the production of more saliva.

To protect against tooth decay and gum disease, look to ingredients like clove oil, cinnamon oil or liquorice root powder. If you want stronger gums and better gum health in general, add some triphala or neem powder to your oil.

Try out different oils or oil-based mouthwashes to find which one suits you best. You want your choice of oil or mouthwash to motivate you to oil pull every day.

'Okay,' Jaya said, 'I should oil pull after I've brushed, flossed and cleaned my tongue, right?'

'Yes, try to make this a daily habit. If you have a cough, though, I don't recommend it. If you do unexpectedly have to cough while oil pulling, spit out the oil immediately so you don't swallow or inhale the oil.'

I also tell my patients that if they can't breathe through their nose, they may need to spit out the oil sooner and repeat swishing with new oil. And if they clench or grind their teeth, they may have to shorten the time they oil pull because sore, fatigued jaw muscles can become even more tired with prolonged oil pulling.

'So how exactly do I do this?' Jaya asked.

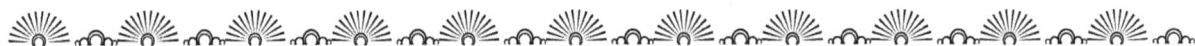

HOW TO OIL PULL

- Place one teaspoon of oil in your mouth. If the oil you're using is in its solid form, don't worry, as it will melt within a few seconds of being inside your mouth.
- Try to swish for as long as you feel comfortable, which could be anywhere from five to twenty minutes. When I say 'swish', I mean suck the oil between your teeth and 'chew' it. Saliva will start to fill your mouth and it will mix with the oil. Take care to avoid swallowing the oil, as it will contain bacteria, toxins and dead cells.

- When you're finished, spit the oil out into the toilet bowl, the garbage or a garden bed. Don't spit the oil into the sink as it could clog the pipes.

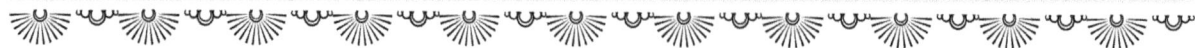

Wash Your Mouth throughout the Day, the Easy Way

'As you go through your day,' I told Jaya, 'a great way to cleanse your mouth and keep your breath fresh is to sip on warm herbal teas.'

Drinking herbal tea is a great way to stay hydrated, nurture a vibrant Agni and allow the mouth to be bathed in the healing properties of plant medicines. The warmth of the tea promotes blood flow to the mouth, which in turn increases absorption of the beneficial herbs into both the mouth and body.

'I love herbal teas. My mother does too. I've been drinking them all my life. The one you served me in the waiting room was delicious.'

'Thank you. That's my Anokhi Veda Ayurvedic blend of organic tulsi, moringa and sweet passionfruit. I formulated it with oral health in mind. These herbs of ancient India are antibacterial and help maintain a balanced microbiome.

'Tulsi is also an adaptogen, which means it's great for managing stress. Moringa is rich in calcium and nourishes the teeth. It's a tea to calm and heal!

'Other teas known for their healing properties include liquorice, mint, fennel, clove, cinnamon and cardamom.'

'That's inspiring,' Jaya said. 'I'm going to set up a tea collection now that I know they have so many benefits.'

Closing the Day: Your Nighttime Ritual

In the chapter 'Stressed-Out Mouth', I mentioned that in Ayurveda, the practices performed after sunset are called Ratricharya. Cleaning your mouth as part of your night routine is as important as it is in the morning. Because the natural cleansing action of saliva slows down during sleep, it's important to remove food particles, plaque and bacteria that have accumulated in the mouth throughout the day.

'I recommend you follow the same routine in the morning and at night, Jaya,' I said.

'That would be good,' she said, 'because I'm studying *and* working part-time. I won't remember what to do when.'

'You won't have to,' I said. 'And you can skip looking at your tongue at night. Just brush your teeth, clean between them, clean your tongue and swish with an oil-based mouthwash.'

'I can't wait to get started,' Jaya said.

'It's more like a meaningful ritual,' I said. 'A

simple, easy one that doesn't take much time but that enhances your health in so many ways.

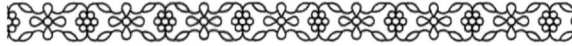

> Cleaning your mouth as part of your night routine is as important as it is in the morning.

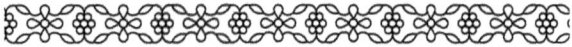

'You're off to such a good start, Jaya,' I said. 'I'll see you at your next check-up.'

Six months later, I saw Jaya again. She now clearly understands when, how and in which order to clean her mouth. She's using her copper tongue cleaner every day. And, she's swapped her plastic toothbrush for a bamboo one and her whitening toothpaste for an Ayurvedic one containing more natural ingredients like clove, bentonite clay and hydroxyapatite.

'I love the flavours of the toothpaste and oil mouthwash. My mouth feels so clean and fresh, and my food even tastes better.'

Jaya is now careful to rinse her mouth after drinking lemon water and enjoys sipping the tulsi and moringa tea throughout the day.

'I love all this,' she said. 'I never knew going to the dentist could be so much fun.'

We've ignited Jaya's passion by turning her routine into a ritual.

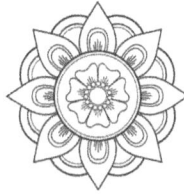

IF IT'S IN YOUR MOUTH, IT'S IN YOUR BODY

My Wish for You

I hope that reading this book has transformed your view of dental health from a mundane, possibly intimidating topic into a gateway to overall wellbeing.

Rather than viewing dentistry as a mechanical process for repairing or enhancing the appearance of your teeth, you now recognise the wisdom and potential that taking care of your mouth holds.

Whether you're concerned about gum disease, tooth decay or grinding, or simply looking for ways to integrate holistic practices into your dental care, I hope you've found information that is helpful and has sent you on your way with an understanding that your mouth and body are one. May you find ways to heal both.

With self-awareness comes self-healing. You can take care of your teeth, gums and oral microbiome in such simple ways, ways Ayurveda has known for thousands of years. Please treasure this ancient wisdom handed down to me and now shared with you. Carry it forward into your life. Incorporate the power of nature, plant medicine and Ayurvedic practices to enhance your wellbeing, just as my grandmother did.

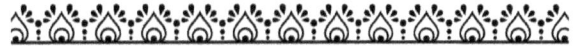

> You can take care of your teeth, gums and oral microbiome in such simple ways, ways Ayurveda has known for thousands of years.

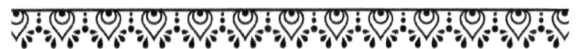

As I was in the final stages of writing this book

and verifying facts with family members, I came across a revelation about Mumaji I hadn't known before. She had a fascination for new technology and a desire to learn how to use a computer. I had no idea! Here was this wise woman immersed in ancient practices yet always open to the new.

Mumaji's life exemplified the essence of what I have come to understand throughout my career: Integrating ancient knowledge into our lives doesn't mean we have to reject modern advancements. We can hold onto the eternal thread, just as Mumaji did. In fact, in many ways, the medicine of the past has become the medicine of the future.

My hope is that a hundred years from now, the revered knowledge captured in this book will remain. My beloved grandmother would want it that way.

I wish for you *Swasta*, the Sanskrit word for wellness.

Namasté, my friend.

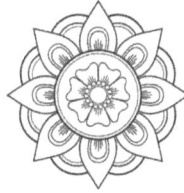

APPENDIX A

Ayurveda Dosha Quiz

Embark on a journey of self-discovery with this Ayurveda Dosha Quiz to reveal the unique balance of energies—Vata, Pitta and Kapha—that define your constitution, your Prakruti.

By answering these questions about your physical traits, mental attributes and lifestyle preferences, you will gain a deeper understanding of your dominant dosha.

Knowledge of your dosha make-up will empower you to make tailored choices in diet, exercise and daily routines to optimise your wellbeing.

Please note that this quiz offers a preliminary insight. For a more comprehensive analysis, please consult with an experienced Ayurvedic practitioner.

To complete the quiz, in each category row ('Physique,' for example) place a tick mark in one of the three boxes across that best describes you or resonates with you. For some categories, it may be helpful to ask someone who knows you well for their opinion, as their perspective could offer greater objectivity.

When you have gone through each profile, add up the tick marks in the columns and place their subtotals in the boxes at the bottom of the profile. After you have completed all five profiles, enter their subtotals into the table at the end of the quiz, then add them together. The highest total number indicates your predominant dosha.

Physical Profile:

Category	Vata	Pitta	Kapha
Physique	thin/slender/delicate frame/long limbs	medium build/muscular/well-defined features	sturdy/solid build/broad shoulders/well-rounded
Physical Activity Level	highly active but variable energy level/prone to restlessness	moderately active/enjoys challenges	steady and consistent/may need motivation to start
Stamina	can be inconsistent and sporadic	moderate/steady	enduring/steady
Tolerance to Pain	low pain threshold/varies/may experience pain differently at different times	medium pain threshold/can tolerate pain but may become irritable	high pain threshold/can endure pain but may take longer to recognise it
Body Weight	low/below average	medium/normal	heavyset/overweight
Skin Type	dry/rough/thin/cold	smooth/warm/prone to redness and acne	moist/thick/oily/cool
Skin Sensitivity	sensitive to windy and cold weather	sensitive to sun and hot weather	sensitive to rain and humid weather
Sweating Patterns	scanty/irregular sweat distribution/may have dry skin even after sweating	profuse/easily breaks into a sweat/may have strong odour	moderate/steady and even sweat distribution/may feel sticky or heavy
Hair	dry/thin/brittle/frizzy	fine/soft/prone to premature greying or thinning	thick/lustrous/prone to oiliness and dandruff

Category	Vata	Pitta	Kapha
Eyes	small or narrow/ nervous/sensitive to dry air/prone to dark circles or puffiness	medium sized/intense and focussed gaze/ sharp vision with sensitivity to light/ prone to redness or inflammation	large and round/ well-lubricated and moist/steady and calm gaze/may have thicker eyelashes and eyebrows
Blinking of Eyes	frequent/irregular/ quick and fluttery/ may blink more when emotional or in dry or windy conditions	moderate/regular and steady/purposeful and focussed/may blink more when exposed to bright lights and screens	slow and deliberate/ steady and rhythmic/ tends to be less frequent/may blink more when exposed to allergens or irritants
Teeth	small with thin enamel/ tendency for irregular alignment-spacing and crowding	medium sized with strong enamel/ tendency for well-aligned and symmetrical teeth	large and strong with thick enamel/compact alignment and possible crowding
Gums	thin/delicate/prone to receding	soft/fleshy/prone to inflammation and redness	thick/sturdy/prone to accumulating plaque
Lip Texture	dry/chapped/thin/ tendency towards cracking	warm/soft/may have reddish or rosy tint/sensitive to sun exposure	moist/well-hydrated/ may appear plump or full/potential for cold sores

Category	Vata	Pitta	Kapha
Cheeks	prominent cheekbones/angular or slightly hollow appearance/potential for uneven skin texture or discolouration/ tendency for dryness and sensitivity	well-defined cheekbones/ balanced and proportionate/ may have rosy or flushed tint/ potential for freckles, sunspots and acne	full and rounded/ may appear plump and well-hydrated/ balanced skin texture/ prone to excess moisture or oiliness
Neck	thin and slender/ potential for stiffness, tension and cracking sounds during movement/prone to knots in muscles	moderate size/prone to heat or redness/ potential for muscles tightness or stiffness	strong and stout/may experience stiffness or heaviness/potential for fluid retention and lymphatic congestion
Chest	thinner and narrower chest/may have prominent collarbones	well-proportioned and balanced/ symmetrical and athletic appearance	well-developed and sturdy/robust and rounded appearance
Abdomen	tendency for narrower or more angular abdomen/may have fluctuations in shape and bloating	generally well-proportioned and balanced/contours might be symmetrical and athletic	well-developed and sturdy/contours might be rounded and robust

Category	Vata	Pitta	Kapha
Hips and Thighs	slim/may vary in shape/fluctuations in weight or muscle tone	moderate and well-proportioned/ muscular definition and symmetry	well-developed and broader hip structure/ thick and well-defined thigh muscles
Joints	tendency towards instability or mobility/ may experience joint discomfort, cracking sounds or stiffness	generally moderate and well-functioning joints/potential for inflammation and swelling	large and sturdy/well-lubricated/potential for fluid retention and puffiness
Nails	dry/brittle/thin/break easily/tendency towards ridges or irregularities	strong/flexible/ pinkish tint/lustrous/ prone to redness around nail bed	thick/smooth/shiny/ hard/tendency towards bacterial or fungal infections
Subtotal			

Diet & Digestion Profile:

Category	Vata	Pitta	Kapha
Appetite	variable and irregular/tendency to get hungry after eating but may also forget to eat/may become full with smaller portions/ prone to digestive sensitivity and discomfort if meals are delayed	generally consistent around regular mealtimes/tends to have strong digestive fire and hunger/may prefer flavourful foods/prone to irritability if meals delayed or skipped	steady and stable/takes longer to feel full due to slower metabolism/ can easily overeat/may not get hungry as frequently
Digestion	variable and irregular/sensitive digestion/gas, bloating and discomfort if meals not taken at regular intervals or incompatible foods consumed	strong and efficient/may experience acid reflux, heartburn or irritability if consuming spicy, acidic or fried foods	slow and heavy/prone to sluggishness and congestion if consuming heavy, oily or sweet foods
Eating Style	fast eater/may rush through meals	moderate eater/enjoys meals but can eat quickly	slow eater/ takes time to savour each bite

Category	Vata	Pitta	Kapha
Food Sensitivities	cold, raw, dry foods/ excess caffeine, carbonated drinks and stimulants	spicy, sour, fried foods/alcohol	heavy, oily, sweet foods/dairy
Digestive Issues	bloating/gas/ irregular digestion/ constipation	acid reflux/heartburn/ inflammation/diarrhoea	sluggish digestion/ heaviness after meals/congestion/ mucous production
Frequency of Thirst	variable/may forget to drink	moderate/frequent	less frequent thirst
Regularity of Bowel Movements	irregular/variable	generally regular	slow/steady
Stools Consistency	dry and hard/low water content	soft and loose/high water content	heavy and dense/oily
Subtotal			

Mental Profile:

Category	Vata	Pitta	Kapha
Speech	quick/talkative/ animated/ may change topics rapidly	clear/articulate/ purposeful/may be assertive or tense	slow/deliberate/may have a calming, soothing quality
Memory	variable/prone to forgetfulness	sharp/focussed/good short-term memory	steady/reliable/good long-term memory
Inquisitiveness	curious and explorative/ seeks variety	intellectually curious/enjoys deep exploration	thoughtful and patient/ seeks understanding over time
Grasping of Ideas	quick to grasp ideas but may have fleeting understanding	sharp and analytical/ grasps ideas with depth	slow and steady/may take time to fully understand but retains well
Mindset	creative and adaptable/can be anxious or fearful	focussed and determined/can become intense or competitive	calm and stable/can resist change or become complacent
Decision Making	quick to decide/ unpredictable/may change mind easily	decisive/logical/can be impatient or forceful	thoughtful/deliberate/may take time to make choices
Enjoyment	creativity/travel/ change/new experiences	challenges/leadership/ intellectual pursuits	stability/comfort/nature/ nurturing activities

Category	Vata	Pitta	Kapha
Sleep	variable sleep patterns/light sleeper/may have difficulty falling asleep	generally sound sleep/ may wake up due to intense dreams or thoughts	deep and long sleep/may have difficulty waking up in the morning
Subtotal			

Behavioural Profile:

Category	Vata	Pitta	Kapha
Work Attitude	self-starter/ creative/adaptable/ may struggle with consistency	driven/goal-oriented/can be competitive or perfectionist	steady/prefers routine/may resist change
Work Style	creative and innovative/speed orientated/can be scattered or disorganised	efficient and focussed/can be intense or impatient	slow and methodical/ once committed, is consistent
Job Performance	fluctuates	consistently progressive	steady and stable

Category	Vata	Pitta	Kapha
Relationship to Money	not very important/ may have fluctuating financial habits/ spends easily	ambitious and focussed on achieving financial success/spends for a purpose	stable and cautious/ values security and savings/spends with difficulty
Confidence Level	timid and variable/ can feel confident one moment and uncertain the next	high outward confidence/ assertive and self-assured	steady, inner confidence/grounded
Social Relations	socialises often without a defined purpose/has a wide circle of friends/ enjoys meeting new people/may have changing social circles	engaging and socialises with a purpose/ prefers a smaller circle of friends/ values quality over quantity/ may become competitive or argumentative	warm and supportive/prefers close-knit and long-lasting relationships/ may have a few but very close friends
Social Attachments	forms attachments quickly/can also detach quickly	forms strong and intense attachments/may struggle to let go	forms deep and en-during attachments/ values stability and loyalty

Category	Vata	Pitta	Kapha
Love Relationships	affectionate and spontaneous/ seeks variety and excitement	passionate and intense/ values depth and connection	stable and nurturing/ seeks comfort and long-lasting bonds
Relationship with Spouse/Partner	clingy/may need grounding and stability	changes slowly/ may need to manage intensity and conflicts	steady and stable/ may need to avoid complacency and encourage growth
Sexual Drive	variable/can be quick and spontaneous but also fickle	intense and passionate/seeks deep connection	slow but sustained interest/values emotional intimacy
Hobbies	creative/writing/ art and exploring new places	competitive/ adventurous/ intellectual and outdoor games	nurturing/ cooking/reading and gardening
Sub total			

Emotional Profile:

Category	Vata	Pitta	Kapha
Presentation of Emotional Disturbance	anxiety/restlessness/ fear/disrupted sleep patterns and insomnia/mood swings and emotional instability	intense/anger/ irritability/frustration/ difficulty letting go of negative emotions	withdrawal/sadness/ depression/lack of motivation/difficulty adapting to change or moving forward

Category	Vata	Pitta	Kapha
Sensitivities	loud noises	bright lights	strong odours
Anger	quick and unstable/ quick to cool down	intense and fiery/can be short-tempered	slow but can hold onto resentment if provoked
Response to Problem	anxious/ overwhelmed/seeks creative solutions	analytical/ determined/seeks logical solutions	takes time to process and respond/seeks stability
When Threatened	may become fearful or scattered/ may seek to escape or avoid	can become intense or defensive/ may seek to confront or assert	may become passive or withdrawn/may seek to protect and preserve
Subtotal			

	Vata	Pitta	Kapha
Physical			
Diet and Digestion			
Mental			
Behavioural			
Emotional			
Total			

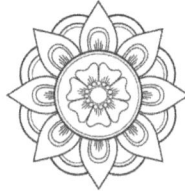

APPENDIX B

Resources

Ayurveda

Frawley, David and Lad, Vasant. *Yoga Of Herbs: An Ayurvedic Guide to Herbal Medicine*. Lotus Brands: Wisconsin, 2001.

Lad, Vasant. *Ayurveda: The Science of Self-Healing*. Lotus Brands: Wisconsin, 1987.

The Complete Book of Ayurvedic Home Remedies: A comprehensive guide to the ancient healing of India. Little Brown: Boston, 2007.

Textbook of Ayurveda: Volume 1 Fundamental Principles of Ayurveda. Ayurvedic Press: North Carolina, 2002.

On the daily routine: https://www.youtube.com/watch?v=PdpjkkaFiIA

Diet and Lifestyle

Anodea, Judith. *Wheels Of Life: User's Guide to the Chakra System*. Llewellyn Worldwide: Minnesota, 1987.

Chopra, Deepak. *Perfect Digestion: The Complete Mind-Body Programme for Overcoming Digestive Disorders*. Random House: London, 2000.

Irani, Farida. *The Magic of Ayurveda Aromatherapy*. 2001.

Matthews, Shaun. *The Art of Balanced Living: The Right Diet and Lifestyle for your Body Type*. Finch Publishing: Sydney, 2015.

Price, Weston. *Nutrition and Physical Degeneration: A Comparison of Primitive and Modern Diets and Their Effects*. Benediction Classics: Oxford, 2010.

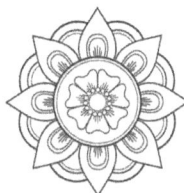

Endnotes

CHAPTER 1

1 Singh, Malvika. (2021). Tulsi: From the Desk of a Periodontist. *CHRISMED Journal of Health and Research*. 8. 3-5. 10.4103/cjhr.cjhr_38_21. https://www.research-gate.net/publication/352509901_Tulsi_From_the_Desk_of_a_Periodontist

2 Syahdiana W, et al. Antibacterial activity of cinnamon ethanol extract (*cinnamomum burmannii*) and its application as a mouthwash to inhibit *streptococcus* growth. 2018 *IOP Conf. Ser.: Earth Environ. Sci.* 130 012049. doi: 10.1088/1755- 1315/130/1/012049.
Gandhi HA, Srilatha KT, Deshmukh S, Venkatesh MP, Das T, Sharieff I. Comparison of Antimicrobial Efficacy of Cinnamon Bark Oil Incorporated and Probiotic Blend Incorporated Mucoadhesive Patch against Salivary *Streptococcus mutans* in Caries Active 7-10-year-old Children: An *In Vivo* Study. *Int J Clin Pediatr Dent.* 2020 Sep-Oct;13(5):543-550. doi: 10.5005/jp-journals-10005-1818. PMID: 33623345; PMCID: PMC7887182. https://www.ncbi.nlm.nih.gov/pmc/articles/PMC7887182/

3 Younis SH, Obeid RF, Ammar MM. Subsurface enamel remineralization by Lyophilized Moringa leaf extract loaded varnish. *Heliyon*. 2020;6(9):e05054. doi: 10.1016/j.heliyon.2020.e05054. PMID: 33015394; PMCID: PMC7522384.

CHAPTER 2

4 Two billion people practice yoga "because it works". UN News. Published June 21, 2016. Accessed July 20, 2022. https://news.un.org/en/audio/2016/06/614172

5 Ginter E, Simko V. New data on harmful effects of trans-fatty acids. *Bratisl Lek Listy*. 2016;117(5):251-3. doi: 10.4149/bll_2016_048. PMID: 27215959.

6 Sharma H, Zhang X, Dwivedi C. The effect of ghee (clarified butter) on serum lipid levels and microsomal lipid peroxidation. *Ayu*. 2010;31(2):134-40. doi: 10.4103/0974-8520.72361. PMID: 22131700;

PMCID: PMC3215354. https://pubmed.ncbi.nlm.nih.gov/22131700/

7 Stoy, S, McMillan, A, Ericsson, AC, Brooks, AE. The effect of physical and psychological stress on the oral microbiome. Frontiers in Psychology. 2023;14. Accessed January 5, 2024. https://www.frontiersin.org/articles/10.3389/fpsyg.2023.1166168.

8 Jaiswal YS, Williams LL. A glimpse of Ayurveda - The forgotten history and principles of Indian tradition-al medicine. *J Tradit Complement Med*. 2016 February 28;7(1):50-53. doi: 10.1016/j.jtcme.2016.02.002. PMID: 28053888; PMCID: PMC5198827.

9 Wacker, M, Holick, M. Sunlight and Vitamin D: A global perspective for health. *Dermato-Endocrinology*. 2013;5(1):51-108. Accessed July 20, 2022. https://www.tandfonline.com/doi/full/10.4161/derm.24494?scroll=top&needAccess=true&role=tab Harvard Health Publishing.

Benefits of moderate sun exposure. Harvard Medical School. Published January 20, 2017. Accessed July 20, 2022. https://www.health.harvard.edu/diseases-and-conditions/benefits-of-moderate-sun-exposure

10 RMIT Online. How having a daily routine can lead to success. RMIT University. Published May 18, 2022. Accessed June 22, 2022. https://online.rmit.edu.au/blog/how-having-daily-routine-can-lead-success

11 Krishnan K, Chen T, Paster BJ. A practical guide to the oral microbiome and its relation to health and disease. *Oral Dis*. 2017;23(3):276-286. doi: 10.1111/odi.12509. Epub 2016 July 4. PMID: 27219464; PMCID: PMC5122475.

12 Li X, Liu Y, Yang X, Li C, Song Z. The oral microbiota: Community composition, influencing factors, patho-genesis, and interventions. *Frontiers in Microbiology*. 2022;13. doi:10.3389/fmicb.2022.895537.

13 Bescos R, Ashworth A, Cutler C, et al. Effects of Chlorhexidine mouthwash on the oral microbiome. *Sci Rep*. 2020;10(1):5254. doi: https://pubmed.ncbi.nlm.nih.gov/32210245/. PMID: 32210245; PMCID: PMC7093448.

14 Blot S. Antiseptic mouthwash, the nitrate-ni-trite-nitric oxide pathway, and hospital mortality: a hy-pothesis generating review. Intensive Care Med. 2021 Jan;47(1):28-38. Accessed January 5, 2024. https://www.ncbi.nlm.nih.gov/pmc/articles/PMC7567004/

15 Wallace RK. The microbiome in health and disease from the perspective of modern medicine and Ayurveda. *Medicina (Kaunas)*. 2020;56(9):462. doi: 10.3390/medicina56090462. PMID: 32932766; PMCID: PMC7559905.

16 Wiertsema SP, van Bergenhenegouwen J, Garssen J, Knippels LMJ. The interplay between the gut microbi-ome and the immune system in the context of infectious diseases throughout life and the role of nutrition in op-timizing treatment strategies. *Nutrients*. 2021;13(3):886. doi: 10.3390/nu13030886. PMID: 33803407; PMCID: PMC8001875.

17 Patel J, Kumar S, Vaidehi Dr, Vinay VR, Sunil Dr, Nikhate P. (2020). An Ayurvedic review of agni and its impact on human health by Dr. Sujit Kumar. *International Journal of Multidisciplinary Research Review*. 2020;4(4): 1920-1923. Accessed January 15, 2023. https://www.researchgate.net/publication/339986978

An Ayurvedic Review of Agni and Its Impact on human health by Dr_Sujit_kumar

18 Wallace RK. The microbiome in health and disease from the perspective of modern medicine and Ayurveda. *Medicina (Kaunas)*. 2020;56(9):462. doi: 10.3390/medicina56090462. PMID: 32932766; PMCID: PMC7559905.

19 Qiang, Z, Zhenyu, Y, Few Wang, et.al. Association between metabolic status and gut microbiome in obese populations. Microbial Genomics. 2021;7(8). https://doi.org/10.1099/mgen.0.000639

20 Cengiz S, Cengiz MI, Saraç YS. Dental erosion caused by gastroesophageal reflux disease: A case report. *Cases J*. 2009;2:8018. doi: 10.4076/1757-1626-2-8018. PMID: 19830044; PMCID: PMC2740145.

21 Kawar N, Park SG, Schwartz JL, et al. Salivary microbiome with gastroesophageal reflux disease and treatment. *Sci Rep*. 2021;11(1):188. doi: 10.1038/s41598-020-80170-y. PMID: 33420219; PMCID: PMC7794605.

22 Jajam M, Bozzolo P, Niklander S. Oral manifestations of gastrointestinal disorders. *J Clin Exp Dent*. 2017;9(10):e1242-e1248. doi: 10.4317/jced.54008. PMID: 29167716; PMCID: PMC5694155.

23 Sensoy I. A review on the food digestion in the digestive tract and the used *in vitro* models. *Curr Res Food Sci*. 2021;4:308- 319. doi: 10.1016/j.crfs.2021.04.004. PMID: 34027433; PMCID: PMC8134715.

24 Yadav, PV. Medical perspective on Ama as per Ayurveda and modern consideration: A review. *Journal of Drug Delivery and Therapeutics*. 10(1-s):205-207. doi:10.22270/jddt.v10i1-s.3861.

25 Komori, E, Kato-Kogoe, N, Imai, Y, et al. Changes in salivary microbiota due to gastric cancer resection and its relation to gastric fluid microbiota. Sci Rep 13, 15863 (2023). https://doi.org/10.1038/s41598-023-43108-8

26 Cherpak CE. Mindful Eating: A review of how the stress-digestion-mindfulness triad may modulate and improve gastrointestinal and digestive function. *Integr Med (Encinitas)*. 2019;18(4):48-53. PMID: 32549835; PMCID: PMC7219460. Accessed March 30, 2023. https://www.ncbi.nlm.nih.gov/pmc/articles/PMC7219460/

CHAPTER 3

27 Ha DH, Spencer JA, Ju X, Do LG. Periodontal diseases in the Australian adult population. *Aust Dent J*. 2020;65 Suppl 1:S52-S58. doi: 10.1111/adj.12765. PMID: 32583592.

28 Darwish, M. (2011). Protective Role of Clove Against Radiation-Induced Oxidative Stress in Rats. https://inis.iaea.org/search/search.aspx?orig_q=RN:44055689

29 Azab, K. S., Mostafa, A. H. A., Ali, E. M., & Abdelaziz, M. A. (2011, November 1). Cinnamon extract ameliorates ionizing radiation-induced cellular injury in rats. Ecotoxicology and Environmental Safety. https://pubmed.ncbi.nlm.nih.gov/21782243/

30 Alsherbiny MA, Abd-Elsalam WH, El Badawy SA, Taher E, et al. Ameliorative and protective effects of ginger and its main constituents against natural, chemical and radiation-induced toxicities: A comprehensive review. *Food Chem Toxicol*. 2019;123:72-97. doi: 10.1016/j.fct.2018.10.048. Epub 2018 October 22. PMID: 30352300.

31 Jagetia GC. Radioprotection and radiosensitization

by curcumin. *Adv Exp Med Biol.* 2007;595:301-20. doi: 10.1007/978-0- 387-46401-5_13. PMID: 17569217.

32 Baliga MS, Rao S, Rai MP, D'souza P. Radio protective effects of the Ayurvedic medicinal plant Ocimum sanctum Linn. (Holy Basil): A memoir. *J Cancer Res Ther.* 2016;12(1):20-7. doi: 10.4103/0973-1482.151422. PMID: 27072205.

33 Kaur S, Arora S, Kaur K, Kumar S. The in vitro antimutagenic activity of Triphala – an Indian herbal drug. *Food Chem Toxicol.* 2002;40(4):527-34. doi: 10.1016/s0278-6915(01)00101-6. PMID: 11893411.

34 McKay DL, Blumberg JB. A review of the bioactivity and potential health benefits of peppermint tea (Mentha piperita L.). *Phytother Res.* 2006 Aug;20(8):619-33. doi: 10.1002/ptr.1936. PMID: 16767798.

35 Karpiński TM, Adamczak A, Ożarowski M. Radioprotective effects of plants from the Lamiaceae family. *Anticancer Agents Med Chem.* 2022;22(1):4-19. doi: 10.2174/1871520620666201029120147. PMID: 33121420.

36 Ryan CS, Kleinberg I. Bacteria in human mouths involved in the production and utilization of hydrogen peroxide. *Arch Oral Biol.* 1995;40(8):753-63. doi: 10.1016/0003-9969(95)00029-o. PMID: 7487577.

37 Panko B. Scientists delve into neanderthal dental plaque to understand how they lived and ate. Smithsonian Magazine. Published March 9, 2017. Accessed February 10, 2023. https://www.smithsonianmag.com/science-nature/delving-neanderthal-dental-plaque-understand-how-they-lived-and-ate-180962449/

38 Adler C, Dobney K, Weyrich L, et al. Sequencing ancient calcified dental plaque shows changes in oral microbiota with dietary shifts of the Neolithic and Industrial revolutions. *Nat Genet.* 2013;45, 450–455 (2013). Accessed November 17, 2022. https://doi.org/10.1038/ng.2536

39 Hadhazy A. A hidden epidemic of shrinking jaws is behind many orthodontic and health issues, Stanford researchers say. Stanford News. Published July 21, 2020. Accessed November 17, 2022. https://news.stanford.edu/2020/07/21/toll-shrinking-jaws-human-health/

40 Shiba, T, Komatsu, K, Sudo, T, et al. Comparison of periodontal bacteria of Edo and modern periods using novel diagnostic approach for periodontitis with micro-CT. Front. Cell. Infect. Microbiol., 20 September 2021;11. | https://doi.org/10.3389/fcimb.2021.723821

41 Olsen I, Yamazaki K. Can oral bacteria affect the microbiome of the gut? *J Oral Microbiol.* 2019 Mar 18;11(1):1586422. doi:10.1080/20002297.2019.1586422. PMID: 30911359; PMCID: PMC6427756. https://www.ncbi.nlm.nih.gov/pmc/articles/PMC6427756/

42 Anand PS, Kamath KP, Anil S. Role of dental plaque, saliva and periodontal disease in *Helicobacter pylori* infection. *World J Gastroenterol.* 2014;20(19):5639-53. doi: 10.3748/wjg.v20.i19.5639. PMID: 24914323; PMCID:PMC4024772.

Jia CL, Jiang GS, Li CH, Li CR. Effect of dental plaque control on infection of *Helicobacter pylori* in gastric mucosa. *J Periodontol.* 2009;80(10):1606-9. https://doi.org/10.1902/jop.2009.090029. PMID: 19792849.

43 Yamazaki, K., & Kamada, N. (2023, November 1). Exploring the oral-gut linkage: Interrelationship between oral and systemic diseases. Mucosal Immunology. https://doi.org/10.1016/j.mucimm.2023.11.006

https://www.sciencedirect.com/science/article/pii/S1933021923000892#:~:text=Oral%20pathobi-onts%20associated%20with%20exacerbation,colitis%20and%20other%20inflammatory%20diseases.

44 Hathaway-Schrader JD, Carson MD, Gerasco JE, et al. Commensal gut bacterium critically regulates alveolar bone homeostasis. *Lab Invest.* 2021;102(4):363-375. doi: https://pubmed.ncbi.nlm.nih.gov/34934182/. Epub ahead of print. PMID: 34934182.

45 Chakraborty A, Anjankar AP. Association of Gastroesophageal Reflux Disease With Dental Erosion. *Cureus.* 2022 Oct 17;14(10):e30381. doi: 10.7759/cureus.30381. PMID: 36407174; PMCID: PMC9667903. https://www.ncbi.nlm.nih.gov/pmc/articles/PMC9667903/

46 Peng, X, Cheng, L, You, Y et al. Oral microbiota in human systematic diseases. *Int J Oral Sci* 14, 14 (2022). https://doi.org/10.1038/s41368-022-00163-7

Gould, S. How bacteria sneak into your blood through your mouth: *Scientific American.* Published January 4, 2012. Accessed August 18, 2023. https://blogs.scientificamerican.com/lab-rat/how-bacteria-sneak-into-your-blood-through-your-mouth/

Fardini, Y, Wang, X, Témoin, S, et al., Y.W. (2011), *Fusobacterium nucleatum* adhesin FadA binds vascular endothelial cadherin and alters endothelial integrity. *Molecular Microbiology*, 82: 1468- 1480. https://doi.org/10.1111/j.1365-2958.2011.07905.x

Patrakka O, Tuomisto S, Ollikainen J, et al. Oral bacterial signatures in cerebral thrombi of patients with acute ischemic stroke treated with thrombectomy. *Journal of the American Heart Association.* 2019;8:e012330. https://doi.org/10.1161/JAHA.119.012330

47 Carrizales-Sepúlveda EF, Ordaz-Farías A, Vera-Pineda R, Flores-Ramírez R. Periodontal disease, systemic inflammation and the risk of cardiovascular disease. *Heart Lung Circ.* 2018;27(11):1327-1334. doi: 10.1016/j.hlc.2018.05.102. Epub 2018 June 2. PMID: 29903685.

48 Gum disease and heart disease: The common thread. Accessed January 5, 2024. https://www.health.harvard.edu/heart-health/gum-disease-and-heart-disease-the-common-thread

49 Sanz M, Marco Del Castillo A, Jepsen S, et al. Periodontitis and cardiovascular diseases: *Consensus report. J Clin Periodontol.* 2020;47(3):268-288. doi: 10.1111/jcpe.13189. Epub 2020 February 3. PMID: 32011025; PMCID: PMC7027895.

50 Research shows if you have gum disease, you're twice as likely to have heart disease. Accessed January 5, 2024. https://www.heartfoundation.org.au/blog/gum-disease-heart-health

51 Byrd KM, Gulati AS. The "gum-gut" axis in inflammatory bowel diseases: a hypothesis-driven review of associations and advances. *Front Immunol.* 2021 February 19;12:620124. doi: 10.3389/fimmu.2021.620124. PMID: 33679761; PMCID: PMC7933581.

52 Ryder MI. *Porphyromonas gingivalis* and Alzheimer disease: Recent findings and potential therapies. *J Periodontol.* 2020;91 Suppl 1(Suppl 1):S45-S49. doi: 10.1002/JPER.20-0104. Epub 2020 August 6. PMID: 32533852; PMCID: PMC7689719.

53 Pazos P, Leira Y, Domínguez C, Pías-Peleteiro JM,

Blanco J, Aldrey JM. Association between periodontal disease and dementia: A literature review. *Neurologia (Engl Ed)*. 2018;33(9):602-613. English, Spanish. doi: 10.1016/j.nrl.2016.07.013. Epub 2016 October 22. PMID: 27780615.

54 Yamaguchi S, Murakami T, Satoh M, et al. Associations of dental health with the progression of hippocampal atrophy in community-dwelling individuals: the ohasama study. *Neurology* July 2023, 10.1212/WNL.0000000000207579; doi: 10.1212/WNL.0000000000207579.

Qi X, Zhu Z, Plassman B, et al. Dose-response meta-analysis on tooth loss with the risk of cognitive impairment and dementia. Published July 8, 2021. Accessed February 19, 2023. https://www.jamda.com/article/S1525-8610(21)00473-4/fulltext

55 Bui FQ, Almeida-da-Silva CLC, Huynh B, et al. Association between periodontal pathogens and systemic disease. *Biomed J*. 2019;42(1):27-35. doi: 10.1016/j.bj.2018.12.001. Epub 2019 March 2. PMID: 30987702; PMCID: PMC6468093.

56 Cheng Z, Meade J, Mankia K, Emery P, Devine DA. Periodontal disease and periodontal bacteria as triggers for rheumatoid arthritis. *Best Pract Res Clin Rheumatol*. 2017;31(1):19-30. doi: 10.1016/j.berh.2017.08.001. Epub 2017 September 1. PMID: 29221594.

57 Preshaw PM, Alba AL, Herrera D, et al. Periodontitis and diabetes: A two-way relationship. *Diabetologia*. 2012;55(1):21-31. doi: 10.1007/s00125-011-2342-y. Epub 2011 November 6. PMID: 22057194; PMCID: PMC3228943.

58 Liccardo D, Cannavo A, Spagnuolo G, et al. Periodontal disease: A risk factor for diabetes and cardiovascular disease. *Int J Mol Sci*. 2019;20(6):1414. doi: 10.3390/ijms20061414. PMID: 30897827; PMCID: PMC6470716.

59 Kim CM, Lee S, Hwang W, et al. Obesity and periodontitis: A systematic review and updated meta-analysis. *Front Endocrinol (Lausanne)*. 2022;13:999455. doi:. PMID: 36353241; PMCID: PMC9637837.

60 Obesity and overweight. World Health Organisation. Published June 9, 2021. Accessed April 17, 2022. https://www.who.int/news-room/fact-sheets/detail/obesity-and-overweight

61 Wahid A, Chaudhry S, Ehsan A, Butt S, Ali Khan A. Bidirectional relationship between chronic kidney disease & periodontal disease. *Pak J Med Sci*. 2013;29(1):211-5. doi: 10.12669/pjms.291.2926. PMID: 24353542; PMCID: PMC3809193. https://www.ncbi.nlm.nih.gov/pmc/articles/PMC3809193/

62 Ricci E, Ciccarelli S, Agnese Mauri P, et al Periodontitis, female fertility and conception (Review). *Biomed Rep*. 2022;17(5):86. doi: 10.3892/br.2022.1569. PMID: 36237287; PMCID: PMC9500491.

Bobetsis YA, Graziani F, Gürsoy M, Madianos PN. Periodontal disease and adverse pregnancy outcomes. *Periodontol 2000*. 2020;83(1):154-174. doi: 10.1111/prd.12294. PMID: 32385871.

63 Tao DY, Zhu JL, Xie CY, et al. Relationship between periodontal disease and male infertility: A case-control study. *Oral Dis*. 2021 Apr;27(3):624-631. doi: 10.1111/odi.13552. Epub 2020 August 31. PMID: 32702140.

64 Wu CD, Darout IA, Skaug N. Chewing sticks: Timeless natural toothbrushes for oral cleansing. *J*

Periodontal Res. 2001;36(5):275-84. doi: https://pubmed. ncbi.nlm.nih.gov/11585114/. PMID: 11585114.

65 Rashid AH, Gul SS, Azeez HA, Azeez SH. Extraction of Cuminum cyminum and Foeniculum vulgare Essential Oils and Their Antibacterial and Antibiofilm Activity against Clinically Isolated Porphyromonas gingivalis and Prevotella intermedia: An In Vitro Study. Applied Sciences. 2023; 13(14):7996. https://doi.org/10.3390/app13147996

66 Badooei F, Imani E, Hosseini-Teshnizi S, Banar M, Memarzade M. Comparison of the effect of ginger and aloe vera mouthwashes on xerostomia in patients with type 2 diabetes: A clinical trial, triple-blind. *Med Oral Patol Oral Cir Bucal*. 2021;26(4):e408-e413. doi: 10.4317/medoral.23998. PMID: 34162822; PMCID: PMC8254880.

Utama-ang N, Sida S, Wanachantararak P, Kawee-ai A. Development of edible Thai rice film fortified with ginger extract using microwave-assisted extraction for oral antimicrobial properties. *Scientific Reports*, 10.1038/s41598-021-94430-y, 11, 1, (2021). Accessed November 10, 2022. https://www.nature.com/articles/s41598-021-94430-y

Saliasi I, Llodra JC, Bravo M, et al. Effect of a toothpaste/mouthwash containing *Carica papaya* leaf extract on interdental gingival bleeding: A randomized controlled trial. *Int J Environ Res Public Health*. 2018;15(12):2660. doi: 10.3390/ijerph15122660. PMID: 30486374; PMCID: PMC6313435.

67 Rowe M, Lawn C, Wilson B. Saliva flow and quality of life in patients with dry mouth using papaya. *Oral Health and Care*. 2018. doi:10.15761/OHC.1000147.

Badooei F, Imani E, Hosseini-Teshnizi S, Banar M, Memarzade M. Comparison of the effect of ginger and aloe vera mouthwashes on xerostomia in patients with type 2 diabetes: A clinical trial, triple-blind. *Med Oral Patol Oral Cir Bucal*. 2021;26(4):e408-e413. doi: 10.4317/medoral.23998. PMID: 34162822; PMCID: PMC8254880.

68 Bhor K, Shetty V, Garcha V, Ambildhok K, Vinay V, Nimbulkar G. Effect of 0.4% Triphala and 0.12% chlorhexidine mouthwash on dental plaque, gingival inflammation, and microbial growth in 14-15-year-old schoolchildren: A randomized controlled clinical trial. *J Indian Soc Periodontol*. 2021;25(6):518-524. doi: 10.4103/jisp.jisp_338_20. Epub 2021 November 1. PMID: 34898918; PMCID: PMC8603804.

69 Vasquez, VG, Guardia, MG. Antibacterial effect of coconut oil (Cocus nucifera) on Streptococcus mutans ATCC 25175: an in vitro study. Int. J. Odontostomat., 15(4):922-927, 2021. Accessed January 5, 2023. https://www.scielo.cl/pdf/ijodontos/v15n4/0718-381X-ijodontos-15-04-922.pdf

70 Tada A, Miura H. The relationship between Vitamin C and periodontal diseases: A systematic review. *Int J Environ Res Public Health*. 2019;16(14):2472. doi:10.3390/ijerph16142472.

71 Pranam S, Palwankar P, Pandey R, Goyal A. Evaluation of efficacy of coenzyme Q10 as an adjunct to nonsurgical periodontal therapy and its effect on crevicular superoxide dismutase in patients with chronic periodontitis. *Eur J Dent*. 2020;14(4):551-557. doi: 10.1055/s-0040-1716596. Epub 2020 September 22. PMID: 32961568; PMCID: PMC7535976.

72 Manthena S, Rao MV, Penubolu LP, Putcha M, Harsha AV. Effectiveness of CoQ10 oral supplements as an adjunct to scaling and root planing in improving periodontal health. *J Clin Diagn Res.* 2015;9(8):ZC26-ZC28. doi:10.7860/JCDR/2015/13486.6291.

Raut CP, Sethi KS, Kohale B, Mamajiwala A, Warang A. Subgingivally delivered coenzyme Q10 in the treatment of chronic periodontitis among smokers: A randomized, controlled clinical study. *J Oral Biol Craniofac Res.* 2019;9(2):204-208. doi:10.1016/j.jobcr.2018.05.005.

73 Allaker RP, Stephen AS. Use of probiotics and oral health. *Curr Oral Health Rep.* 2017;4(4):309-318. doi: 10.1007/s40496- 017-0159-6. Epub 2017 October 19. PMID: 29201598; PMCID: PMC5688201.

74 López-Valverde N, López-Valverde A, Macedo de Sousa B, Rodríguez C, Suárez A, Aragoneses JM. Role of Probiotics in Halitosis of Oral Origin: A Systematic Review and Meta-Analysis of Randomized Clinical Studies. Front Nutr. 2022 Jan 21;8:787908. doi: 10.3389/fnut.2021.787908. PMID: 35127785; PMCID: PMC8813778.

75 Jagelavičienė E, Vaitkevičienė I, Šilingaitė D, Šinkūnaitė E, Daugėlaitė G. The relationship between Vitamin D and periodontal pathology. *Medicina (Kaunas).* 2018;54(3):45. doi: 10.3390/medicina54030045. PMID: 30344276; PMCID: PMC6122115.

Machado V, Lobo S, Proença L, Mendes JJ, Botelho J. Vitamin D and periodontitis: A systematic review and meta-analysis. *Nutrients.* 2020;12(8):2177. doi: 10.3390/nu12082177. PMID: 32708032; PMCID: PMC7468917.

76 Sizar O, Khare S, Goyal A, et al. *Vitamin D deficiency.* StatPearls Publishing; 2023. Updated 2023 February 19. Accessed June 18, 2023. https://www.ncbi.nlm.nih.gov/books/NBK532266/

Machado V, Lobo S, Proença L, Mendes JJ, Botelho J. Vitamin D and periodontitis: A systematic review and meta-analysis. *Nutrients.* 2020;12(8):2177. doi: 10.3390/nu12082177. PMID: 32708032; PMCID: PMC7468917.

77 Kruse AB, Kowalski CD, Leuthold S, Vach K, Ratka-Krüger P, Woelber JP. What is the impact of the adjunctive use of omega-3 fatty acids in the treatment of periodontitis? A systematic review and meta-analysis. *Lipids Health Dis.* 2020;19(1):100. doi: 10.1186/s12944-020-01267-x. PMID: 32438906; PMCID: PMC7240972.

Kujur SK, Goswami V, Nikunj AM, Singh G, Bandhe S, Ghritlahre H. Efficacy of omega 3 fatty acid as an adjunct in the management of chronic periodontitis: A randomized controlled trial. *Indian J Dent Res.* 2020;31(2):229-235. doi: 10.4103/ijdr.IJDR_647_18. PMID: 32436902.

Elgendy EA, Kazem HH. Effect of omega-3 fatty acids on chronic periodontitis patients in postmenopausal women: A randomised controlled clinical study. *Oral Health Prev Dent.* 2018;16(4):327-332. doi: 10.3290/j.ohpd.a40957. PMID: 30175329.

78 Uwitonze AM, Ojeh N, Murererehe J, Atfi A, Razzaque MS. Zinc Adequacy Is Essential for the Maintenance of Optimal Oral Health. Nutrients. 2020 Mar 30;12(4):949. doi: 10.3390/nu12040949. PMID: 32235426; PMCID: PMC7230687.

CHAPTER 4

79 Miller WD. *Micro-Organisms of the Human Mouth*. Philadelphia, Pa, USA: The S. S. White Dental Manufacturing; 1890. Reprint Creative Media Partners, LLC, 2018.

80 Loesche WJ. Microbiology of dental decay and periodontal disease. In: Baron S, ed. *Medical Microbiology*. 4th edition. Galveston (TX): University of Texas Medical Branch at Galveston; 1996. Chapter 99. Accessed April 17, 2023. https://www.ncbi.nlm.nih.gov/books/NBK8259/

81 Sugars and dental caries. World Health Organisation. Published November 9, 2017. Accessed September 19, 2022. https://www.who.int/news-room/fact-sheets/detail/sugars-and-dental-caries

82 About oral health. FDI World Dental Federation. Accessed June 15, 2023. https://www.fdiworlddental.org/key-facts-about-oral-health

83 Price, Weston. Nutrition and Physical Degeneration: *A Comparison of Primitive and Modern Diets and Their Effects*. Benediction Classics: Oxford, 2010.

84 Lin S. Vitamin A for healthy teeth. Accessed June 15, 2023. https://www.drstevenlin.com/vitamin-a-for-teeth/

85 Botelho J, Machado V, Proença L, Delgado AS, Mendes JJ. Vitamin D deficiency and oral health: A comprehensive review. Nutrients. 2020;12(5):1471. doi: 10.3390/nu12051471. PMID: 32438644; PMCID: PMC7285165.

86 Booth SL, Broe KE, Gagnon DR, et al. Vitamin K intake and bone mineral density in women and men. *Am J Clin Nutr*. 2003;77(2):512-6. doi: 10.1093/ajcn/77.2.512. PMID: 12540415.

87 Rios D, Boteon AP, Lira Di Leone CC, et al. Vitamin E: A potential preventive approach against dental erosion – An in vitro short-term erosive study. *Journal of Dentistry*. 2021;113, 103781, ISSN 0300-5712. https://doi.org/10.1016/j.jdent.2021.103781

88 Zhang M, Wang Y, Zhao X, Liu C, Wang B, Zhou J. Mechanistic basis and preliminary practice of butyric acid and butyrate sodium to mitigate gut inflammatory diseases: A comprehensive review. *Nutr Res*. 2021;95:1-18. doi: 10.1016/j.nutres.2021.08.007. Epub 2021 September 9. PMID: 34757305.

89 Chinnadurai K, Kanwal HK, Tyagi AK, Stanton C, Ross P. High conjugated linoleic acid enriched ghee (clarified butter) increases the antioxidant and antiatherogenic potency in female Wistar rats. *Lipids Health Dis*. 2013;12:121. doi: 10.1186/1476-511X-12-121. PMID: 23923985; PMCID: PMC3766171.

90 Watras AC, Buchholz AC, Close RN, Zhang Z, Schoeller DA. The role of conjugated linoleic acid in reducing body fat and preventing holiday weight gain. *Int J Obes (Lond)*. 2007;31(3):481-7. doi: 10.1038/sj.ijo.0803437. Epub 2006 August 22. PMID: 16924272.

91 Steinman R, Leonora J. Relationship of fluid transport through the dentin to the incidence of dental caries. Accessed August 18, 2023. https://www.dr-jacques-imbeau.com/PDF/Dentinal%20fluid%20transport%20and%20caries.pdf

92 Lolayekar NV, Kadkhodayan SS. Estimation of salivary pH and viability of *Streptococcus mutans* on chewing of Tulsi leaves in children. *J Indian Soc Pedod Prev Dent*. 2019;37(1):87-91. doi: 10.4103/JISPPD.JISPPD_91_17. PMID: 30804313.

93 Vaillancourt K, LeBel G, Pellerin G, Ben Lagha A, Grenier D. Effects of the licorice isoflavans licoricidin and glabridin on the growth, adherence properties, and acid production of *streptococcus mutans*, and assessment of their biocompatibility. *Antibiotics (Basel)*. 2021;10(2):163. doi: 10.3390/antibiotics10020163. PMID: 33562595; PMCID: PMC7915699.

94 Chanthaboury M, Choonharuangdej S, Shrestha B, Srithavaj T. Antimicrobial properties of *Ocimum* species: an *in vitro* study. *J Int Soc Prev Community Dent*. 2022;12(6):596-602. doi: 10.4103/jispcd. JISPCD_155_22. PMID: 36777016; PMCID: PMC9912833.

95 Wiwattanarattanabut K, Choonharuangdej S, Srithavaj T. In vitro anti-cariogenic plaque effects of essential oils extracted from culinary herbs. *J Clin Diagn Res*. 2017;11(9):DC30-DC35. doi: 10.7860/ JCDR/2017/28327.10668. Epub 2017 September 1. PMID: 29207708; PMCID: PMC5713730.

Manohar R, Ganesh A, Abbyramy N, Abinaya R, Balaji SK, Priya SB. The effect of fennel seeds on pH of saliva - A clinical study. *Indian J Dent Res*. 2020;31(6):921-923. doi: 10.4103/ijdr.IJDR_185_19. PMID: 33753665.

96 Karimi N, Jabbari V, Nazemi A, et al. Thymol, cardamom and lactobacillus plantarum nanoparticles as a functional candy with high protection against streptococcus mutans and tooth decay. *Microb Pathog*. 2020;148:104481. doi: 10.1016/j.micpath.2020.104481. Epub 2020 September 8. PMID: 32916244.

Aneja K R, Joshi R. Antimicrobial activity of amomum subulatum and elettaria cardamomum against dental caries causing microorganisms. *Ethnobotanical Leaflets*. 2009;2009(7), Article 3. Accessed June 18, 2023.

https://opensiuc.lib.siu.edu/ebl/vol2009/iss7/3/ Swathi V, Rekha R, Abhishek JHA, Radha G, Pallavi SK, Praveen G. Effect of chewing fennel and cardamom seeds on dental plaque and salivary pH – A randomized controlled trial. *IJPSR*. 2015;7(1):406-12. doi:10.13040/ IJPSR.0975-8232.7(1).406-12

97 Younis SH, Obeid RF, Ammar MM. Subsurface enamel remineralization by lyophilized moringa leaf extract loaded varnish. *Heliyon*. 2020;6(9):e05054. doi: 10.1016/j.heliyon.2020.e05054. PMID: 33015394; PMCID: PMC7522384.

98 Utama-ang N, Sida S, Wanachantararak P, Kaweeai A. Development of edible Thai rice film fortified with ginger extract using microwave-assisted extraction for oral antimicrobial properties, Scientific Reports, 10.1038/s41598-021-94430-y, 11, 1, (2021). Accessed June 20, 2023. https://onlinelibrary.wiley.com/doi/ abs/10.1002/9781119618973.ch21

99 Salli K, Lehtinen MJ, Tiihonen K, Ouwehand AC. Xylitol's health benefits beyond dental health: A comprehensive review. *Nutrients*. 2019;11(8):1813. doi: 10.3390/nu11081813. PMID: 31390800; PMCID: PMC6723878.

100 Bossù M, Saccucci M, Salucci A, et al. Enamel remineralization and repair results of Biomimetic Hydroxyapatite toothpaste on deciduous teeth: An effective option to fluoride toothpaste. *J Nanobiotechnology*. 2019;17(1):17. doi: 10.1186/s12951-019-0454- 6. PMID: 30683113; PMCID: PMC6346538.

101 Amaechi BT, AbdulAzees PA, Alshareif DO et al. Comparative efficacy of a hydroxyapatite and a fluoride

toothpaste for prevention and remineralization of dental caries in children. *BDJ Open*. 2019;5(18). https://doi.org/10.1038/s41405-019-0026-8

102 Strunecka A, Strunecky O. Mechanisms of Fluoride Toxicity: From Enzymes to Underlying Integrative Networks. Applied Sciences. 2020; 10(20):7100. https://doi.org/10.3390/app10207100

103 Jiang Y, Guo X, Sun Q, Shan Z, Teng W. Effects of excess fluoride and iodide on thyroid function and morphology. *Biol Trace Elem Res*. 2016;170(2):382-9. doi: 10.1007/s12011-015-0479-0. Epub 2015 August 29. PMID: 26319807.

104 Luke J. Fluoride deposition in the aged human pineal gland. *Caries Res*. 2001;35(2):125-8. doi: 10.1159/000047443. PMID: 11275672.

105 Nakamoto T, Rawls HR. Fluoride exposure in early life as the possible root cause of disease in later life. *J Clin Pediatr Dent*. 2018;42(5):325-330. doi: 10.17796/1053-4625-42.5.1. Epub 2018 May 15. PMID: 29763350.

106 Peckham, S, Awofeso, N. Water Fluoridation: A Critical Review of the Physiological Effects of Ingested Fluoride as a Public Health Intervention. The Scientific World Journal, 2014; Article ID 293019. https://doi.org/10.1155/2014/293019

107 Madhusudhan N, Basha PM, Rai P, Ahmed F, Prasad GR. Effect of maternal fluoride exposure on developing CNS of rats: protective role of Aloe vera, Curcuma longa and Ocimum sanctum. *Indian J Exp Biol*. 2010;48(8):830-6. PMID: 21341542. Accessed March 20, 2023. https://pubmed.ncbi.nlm.nih.gov/21341542/ Sharma C, Suhalka P, Sukhwal P, Jaiswal N, Bhatnagar M. Curcumin attenuates neurotoxicity induced by fluoride:

An in vivo evidence. *Pharmacogn Mag*. 2014;10(37):61-5. doi: 10.4103/0973-1296.126663. PMID: 24696547; PMCID: PMC3969660.

108 Williams LB, Haydel SE. Evaluation of the medicinal use of clay minerals as antibacterial agents. *Int Geol Rev*. 2010;52(7/8):745-770. doi: 10.1080/00206811003679737. PMID: 20640226; PMCID: PMC2904249.

109 Moosavi M. Bentonite clay as a natural remedy: A brief review. *Iran J Public Health*. 2017;46(9):1176-1183. PMID: 29026782; PMCID: PMC5632318. Accessed July 17, 2022. https://www.ncbi.nlm.nih.gov/pmc/articles/PMC5632318/

CHAPTER 5

110 Emodi-Perlman A, Eli I, Smardz J, et al. Temporomandibular disorders and bruxism outbreak as a possible factor of orofacial pain worsening during the covid-19 pandemic—concomitant research in two countries. *Journal of Clinical Medicine*. 2020;9(10): 3250. Accessed April 5, 2022. https://doi.org/10.3390/jcm9103250

111 Science Reference Section, Library of Congress. Everyday Mysteries: What is the strongest muscle in the human body? Library of Congress. Published November 19, 2019. Accessed April 5, 2022. https://www.loc.gov/everyday-mysteries/biology-and-human-anatomy/item/what-is-the-strongest-muscle-in-the-human-body/

112 Hilton TJ, Funkhouser E, Ferracane JL, et al.; National Dental Practice-Based Research Network Collaborative Group. Correlation between symptoms and external characteristics of cracked teeth: Findings

from The National Dental Practice-Based Research Network. *J Am Dent Assoc.* 2017 Apr;148(4):246-256.e1. doi: 10.1016/j.adaj.2016.12.023. Epub 2017 February 2. PMID: 28160942; PMCID: PMC5376224.

113 Bulanda S, Ilczuk-Rypuła D, Nitecka-Buchta A, Nowak Z, Baron S, Postek-Stefańska L. Sleep bruxism in children: etiology, diagnosis, and treatment – A literature review. *Int J Environ Res Public Health.* 2021;18(18):9544. doi: 10.3390/ijerph18189544. PMID: 34574467; PMCID: PMC8471284.

114 Hook M. Dentists say teeth grinding has increased during pandemic. ABC News. Published November 22, 2021. Updated November 22, 2021. Accessed April 5, 2022. https://www.abc.net.au/news/2021-11-22/dentists-report-teeth-grinding-increase-during-pandemic/100638656

115 Sutin AR, Terracciano A, Ferrucci L, Costa PT Jr. Teeth grinding: Is emotional stability related to bruxism? *J Res Pers.* 2010;44(3):402-405. doi: 10.1016/j.jrp.2010.03.006. PMID: 20835403; PMCID: PMC2934876.

116 Kolak V, Pavlovic M, Aleksic E, Biocanin V, Gajic M, Nikitovic A, Lalovic M, Melih I, Pesic D. Probable Bruxism and Psychological Issues among Dental Students in Serbia during the COVID-19 Pandemic. Int J Environ Res Public Health. 2022 June 23;19(13):7729. doi: 10.3390/ijerph19137729. PMID: 35805387; PMCID: PMC9266173.

117 Chemelo VDS, Né YGS, Frazão DR, de Souza-Rodrigues RD, Fagundes NCF, Magno MB, da Silva CMT, Maia LC, Lima RR. Is There Association Between Stress and Bruxism? A Systematic Review and Meta-Analysis. Front Neurol. 2020 December 7;11:590779. doi: 10.3389/fneur.2020.590779. PMID: 33424744; PMCID: PMC7793806.

118 Bucci C, Amato M, Zingone F, Caggiano M, Iovino P, Ciacci C. Prevalence of sleep bruxism in IBD patients and its correlation to other dental disorders and quality of life. *Gastroenterology Research and Practice.* 2018;Vol. 2018, Article ID 7274318, 5 pages. https://doi.org/10.1155/2018/7274318

119 Li Y, Yu F, Niu L, et al. Associations among bruxism, gastroesophageal reflux disease, and tooth wear. *Journal of Clinical Medicine.* 2018;7(11): 417. https://doi.org/10.3390/jcm7110417

120 Alkhatatbeh MJ, Hmoud ZL, Abdul-Razzak KK, Alem EM. Self-reported sleep bruxism is associated with Vitamin D deficiency and low dietary calcium intake: A case-control study. *BMC Oral Health.* 2021;21(1):21. doi: 10.1186/s12903-020-01349-3. PMID: 33413308; PMCID: PMC7792220.

Pavlou IA, Spandidos DA, Zoumpourlis V, Adamaki M. Nutrient insufficiencies and deficiencies involved in the pathogenesis of bruxism (Review). *Exp Ther Med.* 2023 Oct 19;26(6):563. doi: 10.3892/etm.2023.12262. PMID: 37954114; PMCID: PMC10632959.

121 Teoh L, Moses G, Duma SR, Fung VS. Drug-induced bruxism. *Aust Prescr.* 2019;42:121. https://doi.org/10.18773/austprescr.2019.048

122 Bertazzo-Silveira E, Kruger CM, Porto De Toledo I, et al. Association between sleep bruxism and alcohol, caffeine, tobacco, and drug abuse: A systematic review. J Am Dent Assoc. 2016 Nov;147(11):859-866.e4. doi: 10.1016/j.adaj.2016.06.014. Epub 2016 Aug

10. PMID: 27522154. https://pubmed.ncbi.nlm.nih.gov/27522154/

123 Martynowicz H, Gac P, Brzecka A, et al. The Relationship between Sleep Bruxism and Obstructive Sleep Apnea Based on Polysomnographic Findings. J Clin Med. 2019 Oct 11;8(10):1653. doi: 10.3390/jcm8101653. PMID: 31614526; PMCID: PMC6832407.

124 Michalek-Zrabkowska M, Wieckiewicz M, Macek P, et al. The Relationship between Simple Snoring and Sleep Bruxism: A Polysomnographic Study. Int J Environ Res Public Health. 2020 Dec 2;17(23):8960. doi: 10.3390/ijerph17238960. PMID: 33276496; PMCID: PMC7731201.

125 Gilani AH, Jabeen Q, Khan AU, Shah AJ. Gut modulatory, blood pressure lowering, diuretic and sedative activities of cardamom. J Ethnopharmacol. 2008;115(3):463-72. doi: 10.1016/j.jep.2007.10.015. Epub 2007 October 22. PMID: 18037596.

126 Kulkarni SK, Bhutani MK, Bishnoi M. Antidepressant activity of curcumin: Involvement of serotonin and dopamine system. Psychopharmacology. 2008;201, 435-442. https://doi.org/10.1007/s00213-008-1300-y

127 Muchtaridi M, Subarnas A, Apriyantono A, Mustarichie R. Identification of compounds in the essential oil of nutmeg seeds (Myristica fragrans Houtt.) that inhibit locomotor activity in mice. Int J Mol Sci. 2010;11(11):4771-81. doi: 10.3390/ijms11114771. PMID: 21151471; PMCID: PMC3000115.

128 Jitomir J, Willoughby DS. Cassia cinnamon for the attenuation of glucose intolerance and insulin resistance resulting from sleep loss. J Med Food. 2009;12(3):467-72. doi: 10.1089/jmf.2008.0128. PMID: 19627193.

129 Pachikian BD, Copine S, Suchareau M, Deldicque L. Effects of saffron extract on sleep quality: A randomized double-blind controlled clinical trial. Nutrients. 2021;13(5):1473. doi: 10.3390/nu13051473. PMID: 33925432; PMCID: PMC8145009.

130 Cheah KL, Norhayati MN, Husniati Yaacob L, Abdul Rahman R. Effect of Ashwagandha (Withania somnifera) extract on sleep: A systematic review and meta-analysis. PLoS One. 2021 Sep 24;16(9):e0257843. doi: 10.1371/journal.pone.0257843. PMID: 34559859; PMCID: PMC8462692. https://www.ncbi.nlm.nih.gov/pmc/articles/PMC8462692/

131 Tiwari, Dr & Talreja, S. (2020). Insomnia: A Study on Sleeping Disorder with the Reference of Ayurvedic Herbs. Journal of Pharmaceutical Sciences and Research. 12. 1375-1379. https://www.researchgate.net/publication/346475716_Insomnia_A_Study_on_Sleeping_Disorder_with_the_Reference_of_Ayurvedic_Herbs

132 Singh N, Garg M, Prajapati P, et al. Adaptogenic property of Asparagus racemosus: Future trends and prospects. Heliyon. 2023 Apr 1;9(4):e14932. doi: 10.1016/j.heliyon.2023.e14932. PMID: 37095959; PMCID: PMC10121633. https://www.ncbi.nlm.nih.gov/pmc/articles/PMC10121633/

133 Pereira N, Naufel MF, Ribeiro EB, Tufik S, Hachul H. Influence of dietary sources of melatonin on sleep quality: A review. J Food Sci. 2020;85(1):5-13. doi: 10.1111/1750-3841.14952. Epub 2019 December 19. PMID: 31856339.

134 Capuano E, Fogliano V. Acrylamide and

5-hydroxymethylfurfural (HMF): A review on metabolism, toxicity, occurrence in food and mitigation strategies. *LWT - Food Science and Technology*. 2011;44(4)793-810, ISSN 0023-6438. https://doi.org/10.1016/j.lwt.2010.11.002

Annapoorani A, Anilakumar KR, Khanum F, Murthy NA, Bawa AS. Studies on the physicochemical characteristics of heated honey, honey mixed with ghee and their food consumption pattern by rats. *Ayu*. 2010;31(2):141-6. doi: 10.4103/0974- 8520.72363. PMID: 22131701; PMCID: PMC3215355.

135 Gandagi N, et al. Role of paada abhyanga in preventive & curative aspect. *International Ayurvedic Medical Journal*. 2017. Accessed May 15, 2023. http://www.iamj.in/posts/2017/images/upload/1317_1323_1.pdf

136 Meth EMS, Brandão LEM, van Egmond LT, et al. A weighted blanket increases pre-sleep salivary concentrations of melatonin in young, healthy adults. *J Sleep Res*. 2023;32(2):e13743. doi: 10.1111/jsr.13743. Epub 2022 October 3. PMID: 36184925.

137 Ekholm B, Spulber S, Adler M. A randomized controlled study of weighted chain blankets for insomnia in psychiatric disorders. *J Clin Sleep Med*. 2020;16(9):1567-1577. doi: 10.5664/jcsm.8636. PMID: 32536366; PMCID: PMC7970589.

CHAPTER 6

138 Fletcher P. African twig brushes offer all-day dental care. Reuters. Updated June 18, 2007. Accessed May 15, 2023. https://www.reuters.com/article/us-africa-toothbrushes-idUSL1487199720070618

139 Torwane NA, Hongal S, Goel P, Chandrashekar BR. Role of Ayurveda in management of oral health. Pharmacogn Rev. 2014;8(15):16-21. doi: 10.4103/0973-7847.125518. PMID: 24600192; PMCID: PMC3931197.

Sharma A, Sankhla B, Parkar SM, Hongal S, Thanveer K, Ajithkrishnan CG. Effect of traditionally used neem and babool chewing stick (datun) on streptococcus mutans: An in-vitro study. *J Clin Diagn Res*. 2014;8(7):ZC15-7. doi: 10.7860/JCDR/2014/9817.4549. Epub 2014 July 20. PMID: 25177629; PMCID: PMC4149135.

Niazi F, Naseem M, Khurshid Z, Zafar MS, Almas K. Role of Salvadora persica chewing stick (miswak): A natural toothbrush for holistic oral health. *Eur J Dent*. 2016;10(2):301-308. doi: 10.4103/1305-7456.178297. PMID: 27095914; PMCID: PMC4813453.

Sidhu P, Shankargouda S, Rath A, Hesarghatta Ramamurthy P, Fernandes B, Kumar Singh A. Therapeutic benefits of liquorice in dentistry. *J Ayurveda Integr Med*. 2020;11(1):82-88. doi: 10.1016/j.jaim.2017.12.004. Epub 2018 November 1. PMID: 30391123; PMCID: PMC7125382.

140 Alli BY, Erinoso OA, Olawuyi AB. Effect of sodium lauryl sulfate on recurrent aphthous stomatitis: A systematic review. *J Oral Pathol Med*. 2019;48(5):358-364. doi: 10.1111/jop.12845. Epub 2019 March 27. PMID: 30839136.

141 Tribble GD, Angelov N, Weltman R, et al. Frequency of tongue cleaning impacts the human tongue microbiome composition and enterosalivary circulation of nitrate. *Front Cell Infect Microbiol*. 2019;9:39. doi: 10.3389/fcimb.2019.00039. PMID: 30881924; PMCID: PMC6406172.

142 Durai Anand T, Pothiraj C, Gopinath RM, Kayalvizhi B. Effect of oil-pulling on dental caries causing bacteria. *Afr J Microbiol Res*. 2008;2(3):63-66. Accessed February 9, 2023. https://academicjournals.org/article/article1380102380_Anand%20et%20al.pdf

143 Amith H, Anil V, Ankola V, Nagesh L. Effect of oil pulling on plaque and gingivitis. *J Oral Health Community Dent*. 2007;1(1):12-18. Accessed February 9, 2023. https://www.oilpullingsecrets.com/OilPullingStudy1.pdf

144 Shanbhag VK. Oil pulling for maintaining oral hygiene - A review. *J Tradit Complement Med*. 2016;7(1):106-109. doi: 10.1016/j.jtcme.2016.05.004. PMID: 28053895; PMCID: PMC5198813.

145 Ibid.

146 Sezgin Y, Memis Ozgul B, Maraş ME, Alptekin NO. Comparison of the plaque regrowth inhibition effects of oil pulling therapy with sesame oil or coconut oil using 4-day plaque regrowth study model: A randomized crossover clinical trial. *Int J Dent Hyg*. 2023;21(1):188-194. doi: 10.1111/idh.12532. Epub 2021 June 28. PMID: 34124840.

147 Tadikonda A, Pentapati KC, Urala AS, Acharya S. Anti-plaque and anti-gingivitis effect of Papain, Bromelain, Miswak and Neem containing dentifrice: A randomized controlled trial. *J Clin Exp Dent*. 2017;9(5):e649-e653. doi: 10.4317/jced.53593. PMID: 28512541; PMCID: PMC5429476.

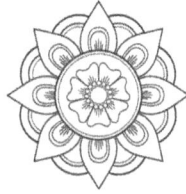

Acknowledgements

To all my patients, who have been my greatest teachers: I am deeply grateful for the privilege of witnessing your journeys. You inspire me beyond words.

To my behind-the-scenes team that helped bring this book to life, let me express my gratitude. Mary Bernstein, thank you for your patience and persistence through the countless edits in our two-year journey together. I couldn't have done it without you. My dear friend Cath Zeltner, you urged me to write a book 16 years ago. At the time, I could only shrug my shoulders and ask, 'What would I write about?' But you wouldn't let it go so easily. When I began to develop my Ayurvedic dental care products, you insisted, 'Now, Aushi, it really is time to write that book.' Thank you for sowing the seed and holding it until I was ready. Kylie Hannaford, many thanks for your beautiful artwork, your vision and your perseverance as we went back and forth with numerous tweaks to the book's design. Once again, you've transformed the essence of my words into art and beauty, as you have so often over the past fifteen years. You revealed my heart's intention before I could perceive it myself. Tom Cronin, thank you for your coaching and guidance and for teaching me so much. Thank you, Dr Shaun Matthews and Farida Irani for your guidance in Ayurveda. I deeply appreciate your gracious willingness to read the manuscript and help me refine its Ayurvedic content.

And finally, to you, dear reader, thank you for being open to exploring a way of wellbeing that extends far beyond your toothbrush.

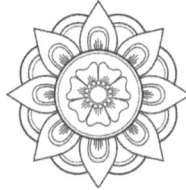

About the Author

Dr Aushi Patel has been a dentist since 1995, having graduated from the prestigious King's College School of Medicine and Dentistry at the University of London. She is the owner of Anokhi Dental, a clinic in the heart of Sydney, Australia, where she integrates her knowledge of the ancient wisdom of Ayurveda with the highest standards of modern dentistry.

Her mission is to elevate awareness about the intimate connection between oral health and overall health. She understands that the mouth serves as the entry point to the digestive system and profoundly influences overall wellbeing.

'It's about much more than teeth,' she says.

Her fresh take on conventional dentistry has established Dr Patel as a visionary thought leader. She believes the time-honoured practices of dental care in traditional cultures have a valuable place in today's world, and through her East-West blend of knowledge, offers an innovative approach to dental health.

In the pages of *Your Healing Mouth,* Dr Patel shares her knowledge and empowers the reader to adopt natural dental care practices that harmoniously meet the demands of modern life.

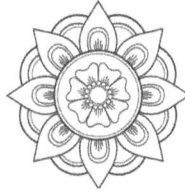

Anokhi Veda Ayurvedic Oral Care

Give your mouth the gift of health with Anokhi Veda Ayurvedic Oral Care. Inspired by ancient Ayurvedic wisdom and created by holistic dentist Dr Aushi Patel, Anokhi Veda offers a collection of gentle, yet effective, oral care products designed to naturally support a healthy mouth.

Anokhi Veda Bamboo Toothbrush

Enjoy a thoughtfully designed toothbrush that combines sustainability with exceptional oral care. Its soft, wavy bristles gently clean your teeth and gums, while the sleek, ergonomic bamboo handle provides a comfortable grip. Make a conscious choice for your dental hygiene and the environment today.

Anokhi Veda Copper Tongue Cleaner

Unlock an ancient secret to oral health with a copper tongue cleaner. This simple yet effective tool gently scrapes away bacteria, toxins and residue from the tongue's surface. Say goodbye to bad breath and hello to a refreshed and healthier mouth with every use.

Anokhi Veda Ayurvedic Toothpaste

Experience the power of a fluoride-free Ayurvedic toothpaste formulated with a traditional blend of clove, cinnamon, liquorice, bentonite clay and nano-hydroxyapatite. This natural, herbal toothpaste supports a balanced oral microbiome while gently cleansing, strengthening and protecting your teeth and gums.

Anokhi Veda Ayurvedic Mouthwash

Enhance your oral care routine with an alcohol--free Ayurvedic mouthwash. Formulated without harsh chemicals, this luxurious blend of coconut oil infused with triphala, papaya, and ginger will keep your mouth feeling fresh and nourished all day. Perfect for a quick swish and oil pulling.

Anokhi Veda Coconut Lime Lip Balm

Pamper your lips with the exquisite essence of this coconut lime lip balm. Enriched with the nourishing properties of jojoba, calendula, copaiba oil and shea butter, this natural balm provides deep hydration, leaving your lips feeling soft, supple and protected.

Anokhi Veda Herbal Tea

Savour the delicious taste of our organic Anokhi Veda herbal tea, a blend designed to support dental health. Tulsi safeguards gums by warding off plaque, while moringa's abundant calcium helps remineralise teeth. With sweet passionfruit undertones, this refreshing tea bathes your mouth in the goodness of healing herbs.

To purchase these products scan the QR code
below or visit
www.anokhiveda.com.au

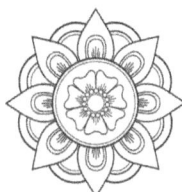

Index

A

Abhyanga 82, 83, 84
acidity 36
acidogenic 50
Acidogenic theory 56
acid reflux 22, 37, 58, 76
Activator X. *See* Vitamin K2
adaptogen 6, 109
adaptogens 81
aerobic bacteria 34
Agni (fire) 19, 20, 22, 23, 25, 53, 58, 109
alcohol 36, 42, 57, 76, 77, 107, 148
alkalinity 36, 102
Alzheimer's disease 39, 40
Ama (undigested food) 20, 22, 23, 95, 104
Anaerobic bacteria 31, 34, 42
anaesthetics 6, 61
Ancient Chinese Medicine 44
angina 100
antidepressant 70, 76
antipsychotics 76
aromatherapy 80
artificial colours 101
artificial flavours 101
artificial intelligence 8
artificial sweeteners 101

Ashwaghanda (Withania somnifera) 81
aspartame 101
atherosclerotic plaques 39
attention deficit hyperactivity disorder (ADHD) 76
autoimmune 36, 40
autoimmune disorders 36
Ayurveda xii, 4, 7, 8, 9, 10, 11, 12, 14, 15, 16, 17, 18, 19, 20, 21, 23, 24, 25, 47, 48, 52, 53, 55, 61, 65, 67, 73, 74, 79, 80, 81, 82, 83, 85, 104, 106, 107, 109, 111
Ayurvedic doshas 12
Ayurvedic medical school 11
Ayurvedic medicine 10, 11, 12, 15, 53, 81, 102, 104
Ayurvedic mouthwash 45
Ayurvedic principle 15
Ayurvedic texts 82
Ayurvedic tradition 21, 93, 98
Ayurvedic wisdom 16, 19, 23, 75
Ayus 8

B

bamboo toothbrush 147
bentonite clay 66, 102, 110
biofilm. *See* plaque
biomimetic. *See* hydroxyapatite
bonding 77
botanicals xiii, 5, 6, 46, 80

Brahmi (Bacopa monnieri) 81
bruxism 73, 75, 76, 79
butyric acid 53
B vitamins 22

C

candidiasis 76
cardamom 44, 46, 58, 81, 82, 109
cardiologist 30, 48
cardiovascular disease 38
carrageenan 101
chai xiii, 15, 32, 44
chakra 77
chiropractor 3, 78
Chronic obstructive pulmonary disease (COPD) 40
cinnamon 5, 32, 43, 44, 46, 61, 66, 81, 82, 102, 108, 109
clenching and grinding 69, 70, 73
clove 61
coconut oil 15, 45, 46, 62, 107
Coenzyme Q10 47
colon cancer 37
constipation 12, 22
copper tongue cleaner 105, 110
cortisol 75
cosmetic service 3
Crohn's disease 22
customised oral care plan 42

D

Datoon (chewing sticks) 97, 98
deep scaling 42
dementia 40
dental apothecary 5
dental care x, 3, 7, 13, 14, 62, 66, 91, 102, 111, 145
dental fluorosis 64
dental health 5, 7, 11, 12, 23, 38, 61, 66, 101, 111

dental patients 12
dental plaque 17, 33, 35, 39, 50
dentinal fluid transport 56
dentine 59, 60, 70, 92
dentist viii, ix, xiii, 3, 4, 7, 13, 20, 29, 31, 33, 38, 50, 51, 56, 59, 60, 61, 62, 65, 73, 78, 91, 93, 96, 110
dentistry x, xi, xiii, 3, 4, 6, 11, 16, 25, 31, 61, 65, 111
dharma 77
diabetes 36, 41
digestive enzymes 23
digestive system 16, 18, 19, 20, 37
Dinacharya 16, 17, 46, 79, 93
diuretic 58
dopamine 76
dosha 12, 13, 14, 15, 23, 75, 82, 83, 86, 113
doshas 12
Dreamtime 9

E

early demineralisation 60
enamel 50, 52, 59, 60, 63, 70, 71, 92
endocrinologist 56
endodontic procedure 59

F

fennel 44
fluoride xi, 37, 42, 49, 63, 64, 65, 66, 148
foaming agents
    Diethanolamine (DEA) 101
    Propylene glycol 101
    Sodium lauryl sulphate (DLS) 101
frankincense 43

G

gandusha 106

gastroesophageal reflux disease 76
gastrointestinal disorders 43
gastrointestinal system 3
ghee 10, 24, 48, 52, 53, 54, 62, 67, 82, 107
ginger 15, 32, 45, 58, 66, 107
gingivitis 30, 32, 33, 38
goitre 52
Golden Milk 33, 81, 82
good health 3, 78, 86
green cardamom pod 44
Gregorian monks 85
grinding xi, 6, 71, 72, 73, 74, 75, 76, 78, 79, 80, 95, 111,
    138
gum disease xi, 5, 6, 11, 22, 31, 32, 36, 38, 39, 40, 41,
    43, 44, 45, 46, 47, 51, 58, 99, 106, 108, 111. *See*
    periodontitis. *See* periodontitis
Gum–Gut Axis 39
gut health 19, 20, 22, 23, 46, 47, 53
gut microbiome 17, 20, 23, 37

H

healthy lifestyle 3
herbal concoctions 4
hippocampal atrophy 40
hippocampus 40
homeopathic drops 100
H. pylori 37
hydrochloric acid 20, 58
hydroxyapatite 63, 64, 66, 102, 110

I

immune system 4, 6, 15, 16, 19, 24, 36, 40, 47, 48
Indian gooseberry. *See* Amla
inflammatory diseases 22, 36, 37, 38
interdental brush 103
intermittent fasting 55

internal equilibrium 14
irritable bowel syndrome 20, 37

J

jaggery 82
Jihva Prakshalana 104

K

kaolin 66
Kapha 12, 13, 14, 83
kavala 106
kidney diseases 43

L

language of ancient India. *See* Sanskrit
lassi 47
leaky gut syndrome 20, 70, 76
lethargic 14
liquorice 44, 46, 58, 66, 98, 102, 108, 109
lung cancer 40

M

magnesium 76
Mahanarayan Thailam 83
malabsorption 22
masseters 69, 71
medicines for healing 4
melatonin 15, 64, 81, 86
microbiome 19, 20, 33, 35, 40, 109
microcosm 12
microorganisms 35
Miller, Dr Willoughby D. 50
mints 22, 44
modernised diet 35

moringa 4, 5, 58, 66, 109, 110, 148
mouthguards 74
mouth ulcers 22, 61, 101
mouthwashes 5, 18, 22, 36, 43, 44, 101, 107, 108
Mukhwas 43
myrrh 43

N

natural teeth cleanser 44
naturopath 3
Neanderthal skulls 35, 65
nervous system 81, 84, 86
nitric oxide 34, 104
non-communicable diseases 50
nutmeg 81, 82
nutrient-dense foods 24, 36

O

obesity 41
oil-based herbal mouthwash 42
oil of eugenol 61
Omega-3 fatty acids 48, 107
Omega-3s 53
oral health x, xi, xiv, 7, 11, 16, 17, 18, 19, 20, 25, 37, 40, 41, 42, 46, 47, 48, 66, 67, 109
oral hygiene 19, 43, 46, 56, 57, 96
oral irrigator 103
oral microbiome 16, 17, 18, 19, 22, 35, 36, 64, 66, 100, 102, 104, 111
oral thrush 61
orthodontic treatment 78
orthopaedics 64
orthopantomogram (OPG) X-ray 33
osteopath 78
oxytocin 86

P

Pada Abhyanga 83
panoramic view 33
papaya 45, 66, 107, 148
parabens 101
parotid glands 56
parsley 43
periodontal disease 31, 32, 33, 36, 38, 40, 41, 47, 48, 79
periodontitis 31, 32, 33, 40, 41
P. Gingivalis 39
pharmaceutical industry 9
pineal gland 15, 64
Pitta 12, 13, 15, 75, 83
Pitta dosha 13, 15, 75
Pitta energy 13
plant medicines 5, 18, 52, 109
plaque 33, 95
Prajnaparadha (crime against wisdom) 21
Prakruti 12
pre-eclampsia 41
preterm birth 41
Price, Dr Weston 38, 51
probiotics 19, 47, 53, 100

R

Ratricharya 16, 79, 109
respiratory infections 43
rheumatoid arthritis 40
root canal treatment. *See* endodontic procedure
root planing 42

S

saccharin 101
sacred Indian herb 4

saffron 81
Sanskrit vii, xi, 8, 15, 20, 43, 46, 77, 81, 82, 85, 97, 106,
    112
Sanskrit chants 85
scurvy 47
seat of the soul 64. *See* pineal gland
seaweed 52
serotonin 86
sesame oil 7, 15, 83, 107
sesame seeds 43, 67
Shatavari (Asparagus racemosus) 81
Shiro Abhyanga 83
sleep hygiene 79
sleep ritual 79
small intestinal bacterial overgrowth (SIBO) 20, 76
sneha 82
sodium lauryl sulphate 101
Solfeggio 85
sorbitol 101
spices and herbs 4, 5, 80, 102
spiritual practice 8
Steinman, Dr Ralph 56
stomach ulcer 30, 37, 39
Streptococcus mutans 50
stressors 74, 86

T

tartar 33, 35, 42
teeth erosion 58
temporomandibular joint (TMJ) 58
testicular dysfunction 41
three pillars of Ayurveda
  Aahar (diet) 10
  Brahmacharya (energy) 10
  Nidra (sleep) 10

thyroid gland 64
titanium dioxide 101
toothache 3, 59, 60, 61
tooth decay 5, 11, 36, 38, 43, 50, 51, 52, 56, 58, 60, 64,
    65, 79, 106, 108, 111
toothpastes 5, 18, 35, 36, 44, 60, 100, 101, 102
traditional Ayurvedic mouthwash 45
traditional medicine 5
triclosan 101
triphala
  amla 45, 46, 47
  bibhitaki 46
  haritaki 46
tulsi 5, 109
tulsi plant xiii, 4
turmeric 32, 33, 46, 61, 62, 65, 81, 82

U

ulcerative colitis 22, 37

V

Vata 12, 13, 14, 75, 83, 86
Vata dosha 12, 13, 75, 86
Vata traits 12, 83
Veda xiii, 8, 109
vitamin A 107
vitamin C 45, 46, 47
vitamin D 15, 48, 52, 76
vitamin E 52
vitamin K2 52

W

wellness xi, xiii, 8, 10, 11, 12, 19, 63, 78, 100, 112

X

X-rays 10, 11, 31, 49, 59

Y

yoga 3, 8, 9, 11, 49, 55, 64, 67
yoga studio 9

www.ingramcontent.com/pod-product-compliance
Lightning Source LLC
Chambersburg PA
CBHW051611030426
42334CB00035B/3486

* 9 7 8 0 6 4 5 9 7 3 0 0 6 *